W9-AOK-611

Individuals with physical disabilities
AN INTRODUCTION FOR EDUCATORS

Individuals with physical disabilities

AN INTRODUCTION FOR EDUCATORS

Gary A. Best, Ph.D.

Professor of Education,
Department of Special Education,
California State University, Los Angeles

with 29 illustrations

The C. V. Mosby Company

Saint Louis   1978

The C. V. Mosby Company
11830 Westline Industrial Drive, St. Louis, Missouri 63141

Library of Congress Cataloging in Publication Data

Best, Gary A., 1939-
    Individuals with physical disabilities.

    Bibliography: p.
    Includes index.
    1. Physically handicapped children.
2. Physically handicapped children—Education.
3. Physically handicapped services. I. Title.
HV903.B47   362.7′8′4   78-18206
ISBN 0-8016-0665-9

TS/CB/B 9 8 7 6 5 4 3 2 1

*. . . if we were intentionally
to neglect the weak and helpless,
it could only be for a contingent benefit
with an overwhelming present evil.*

Charles Darwin: The Descent of Man

FOREWORD

For the teacher entering the field of special education and for teachers and administrators in the regular schools who will have more children with handicaps placed in their schools by provisions of Public Law (PL) 94-142, the Education for all Handicapped Children Act of 1975, this book is informative, practical, and challenging. Increasingly, handicapped children will be educated with children who are not handicapped if they can function satisfactorily in regular classes with supplementary aids and services. The author's broad background in teaching handicapped children, as well as in teaching at the university level, enables him to present the special child with a realism we in the field can appreciate.

The reader will see that the emphasis in this book is on children, not their disabilities. There is no advocacy of any methodology or curriculum; there are no generalizations; rather, children are presented as individuals having feelings and concerns much the same as their counterparts in the regular school.

In the chapter on cerebral palsy, and in the one on musculoskeletal disabilities and other health impairments, the concerns the teacher should have in planning for the physical and educational programs are indicated. A wealth of information has been provided for the educator, paraprofessional, parent, or anyone interested in having a better understanding and knowledge of the various disabilities.

The chapter on postschool and adult alternatives forcefully brings to the attention of professionals in special education the need to question what is or is not being done to prepare our graduates to cope and live as independent, contributing adults. Several articles written by adults with disabilities are presented to illustrate some of their concerns. In reading these articles the reader should gain some insight into and, hopefully, be able to share some of these expressed feelings.

I was greatly impressed by the description of a typical day in the life of John, an elementary school–aged boy with cerebral palsy. As a principal of a special school, I could substitute the name of practically any child in our school, and this narrative would be accurately repeated. We are given a step-by-step, minute-by-minute account. It is truly illustrative of what happens from the time John gets up at 6:00 AM—how this affects the total family routine; his need to be out in front of the house on time to be put on the special lift-gate bus (with its unpredictable mechanical problems and breakdowns); his classroom routine with the use of special equipment shared by several of the children; and the teamwork of the teacher and the classroom aide. The growing sensitivity of a young boy being assisted in the bathroom by female aides is probed; and accounts are given of the recess and lunchtime activities, of going to the therapy department, and, finally, of arriving home at 4:00 PM (if there are no bus problems). It is a very long day for a child.

What are the desirable characteristics of successful special education teachers? What type of training is needed? What are the components that should be included in the university training program? These questions are fully discussed, and I believe that after reading this book, one will not be surprised or overwhelmed at what is required.

Dr. Best shares his feelings about special education when he states: "No one ever said it was going to be easy. But it is fun, and it is rewarding."

Fred S. Lull, *Principal,*
C. Morley Sellery School,
Gardena, California

PREFACE

The underlying aim of this book is to replace the mystique of specialness with something special: interaction with people. False barriers established because of real or perceived differences are stripped away when one becomes intimate with the topic of individuals with disabilities.

The book contains two main sections. Section One identifies and discusses characteristics of disabilities and disability-related services, and Section Two relates primarily to the learning and educational concerns of those with disabilities.

Section One establishes the concept of primacy of the individual over the fact of disability. Although the characteristics of a disability will have a far-reaching impact on the functioning of the individual, the humanistic qualities of being are what is stressed.

Section Two includes discussions of various concepts of learning, approaches to educational placement and practices, and a special section written by and about adults with disabilities. The book concludes with a look at the implications of Public Law (PL) 94-142 and an expression of where those with disabilities are, and ought to be, in today's social structure.

This book is presented as an overview and introduction to the field of physical disabilities. An attempt is made to present materials that will stimulate thought and awareness of the concerns, characteristics, and practices in the field without beating the reader into submission for accepting any one point of view. The individual teacher cannot be all things to all people, and it is in this light that the reader should approach the education of individuals with physical disabilities. No method or technique is applicable to all students. No curriculum is universally appropriate. No teacher is best suited to teach all children. No school can do it all.

When I first began working with children with physical disabilities, I was unaware of myself in terms of my relations with those who were different. In fact, there were no people who were different as far as I was concerned. This sheltered existence was rudely shattered with my first confrontation at a summer camp with a child "who was crippled with polio." How did one talk to someone who is a cripple? Would I be able to accept this really *strange* kid? Talking was never a problem; acceptance was never a problem. The youngster simply said, "Hi there, my name is Johnny." I was lucky. Those six words made the difference. (His name really *was* John.)

This book was written with the hope that someone would read it. The reading will not in any sense compare to "Hi there, my name is Johnny." However, it might provide some insights into what disability and children with disabilities are about.

If it does, we are indebted to many people who have been responsible for much learning.

It is customary to acknowledge in the preface those who have helped in the preparation of a manuscript. Not one to ignore custom, I wish to thank many. Thank you, John, Maria, Jane, Lila, Mom and Dad, Norbert, Dewey, and Mary. Thank you, Greg and George.

And in my affection, Shirley and Joanna know where they belong.

Gary A. Best

CONTENTS

The photographs introducing each chapter are examples of barriers confronted daily by people with physical disabilities. These photographs are courtesy of Carol Stacy and the students and administration of Chandler Tripp School, San Jose, California.

CHARACTERISTICS OF DISABILITIES AND DISABILITY-RELATED SERVICES

1 Introduction

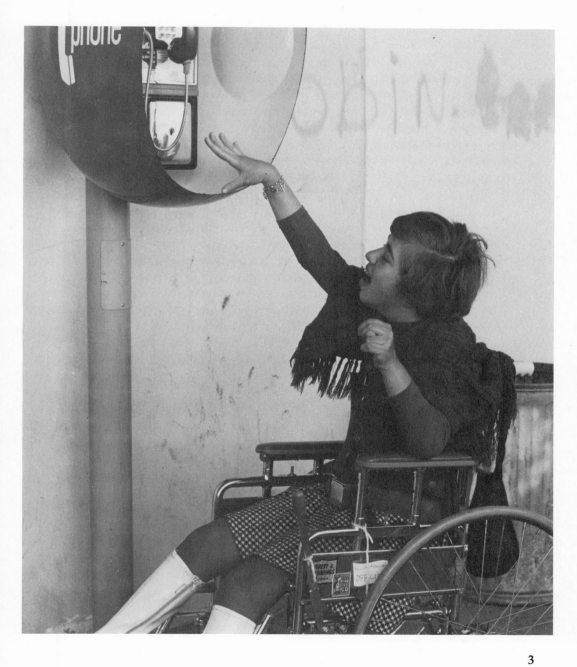

IMPACT OF TERMINOLOGY

For many persons, the concept of physical disabilities has been centered around medical aspects or deviations of the human condition. Such aspects or deviations are referred to as the medical model, and this model has provided the base for descriptions of physical limitations that accompany disability. However, this approach is not always clear or understandable and often is associated with a medicus-mysticus aura. For the teacher, the mystique may be in the realization that one is teaching a *child* or classroom of *children*. This rather simple statement may be crucial in its very simplicity—it may be a philosophical set determining the way in which children, and for that matter, all individuals, are treated in thought and action. The individual, the child, has the preeminent position; the modification of the body, mind, and spirit is secondary. The perspective and philosophical stance of this book is centered on the child: the child with cerebral palsy, the child with a limp, or the child with curly blond hair and blue eyes. Verbalizations may vary, but there is a need to bring the individual to the forefront of consideration. To be considered as an individual is the right and expectation of us all, and this is a right that should be adhered to without fail. The medical model, however, is not itself the culprit. It is only a model behind which it is safe to relate, to act. Any model or set of conditions is a referent from which the whole and not the parts, or even a collection of some of the parts, should be dealt with.

In addition to the medical model, which has been used in describing conditions and in measuring and assessing severity, there are other positions or models that have been utilized in describing children and their particular needs and characteristics. Although not readily recognizable as a model or referent, legislation and its accompanying legal declarations have frequently been responsible for the identification of children, their disabling characteristics, and the methods by which their special needs may be met. The following description, provided by the California Education Code, of "pupils considered physically handicapped" is an example of this method of classification:

> Any pupil who, by reason of a physical impairment, cannot receive the full benefit of ordinary education facilities, shall be considered a physically handicapped individual. . . . Such pupils include the following, as defined by the State Board of Education:
>
> a. The deaf or hard of hearing.
> b. The blind or partially seeing.
> c. Orthopedic or health impaired.
> d. The aphasic.
> e. The speech handicapped.
> f. Other pupils with physical illnesses or physical conditions which make attendance in regular day classes impossible or inadvisable.
> g. Pupils with physical impairments so severe as to require instruction in remedial physical education.
> h. Multihandicapped. (California Education Code, 1976, Section 56701)

The state's administrative guidelines have provided additional definitions by handicap:

> Orthopedic or Other Health Impairment. A minor is orthopedic or other health impaired if a licensed physician and surgeon finds in his diagnosis that the minor has a serious impairment of his locomotion or motor function and that the impairment was caused by crippling due to one of the following:
> 1. Cerebral palsy.
> 2. Poliomyelitis.
> 3. Infection, such as bone and joint tuberculosis and osteomyelitis.
> 4. Birth injury, such as Erb's palsy or fractures.
> 5. Congenital anomalies, such as congenital amputation, clubfoot, congenital dislocations, or spina bifida.
> 6. Trauma, such as amputations, burns, or fractures.
> 7. Tumors, such as bone tumors, or bone cysts.
> 8. Developmental diseases, such as coxa plana or spinal osteochondritis.
> 9. Other conditions, such as fragile bones, muscular atrophy, muscular dystrophy, Perthes' disease, hemophilia, uncontrolled epilepsy, or severe cardiac impairment.
> 10. Drug dependency.
> 11. Some other cause described in the physician's written diagnosis. (California Administrative Code, 1977, Section 3600)

In the same administrative code, the following are presented as part of the population considered eligible for placement in special classes for children with physical disabilities:

> Other Physically Handicapped. A minor is "other physically handicapped" if he comes within either of the following descriptions:
> 1. He has a physical illness or physical condition which makes attendance in regular day classes impossible or inadvisable.
> 2. He has a physical impairment so severe as to require instruction in remedial . . . physical education. (California Administrative Code, 1977, Section 3600)

The first of these legislative classifications seems almost unmanageable in its scope. However, when each of the "physical handicaps" is further defined for administrative implementation, it becomes clearer as to what types of disability would be found in a classroom for the physically disabled. And yet, the ambiguities of the definitions are great. The point at which a child with a physical impairment "cannot receive the full benefit of ordinary education facilities" is so vague as to be capricious. The weight of the burden of definition may fall on the teacher of the regular class because of the system or teacher's inability or unwillingness to accommodate in the class educationally or in any other way, the child with a disability. On the other hand, a child may be functioning very well academically and/or socially and still have difficulty attending a regular school because of limited access to the school building or classrooms. The difficulty, is in this case, based on the architectural features of the building rather than on the competence or abilities of either the child or the teacher.

Legislative codes and definitions concerning special education services for children with special needs often seem to deal with a specified medical diagnosis or condition based on circumstantial phenomena. What may seem to be the basis for providing education to children with special needs has, in effect, been an instrument for excluding children from educational settings that may have provided them with the best educational forum. Reynolds and Balow (1972) have suggested that the legislative structure that is so much a part of educational life, if not of the educational process, is reflected in codification such as that cited on pp. 4-5: categories. According to these authors, such categorical listings do little more than identify the presence of "surface variables," variables that indicate the existence of a condition but are not concerned with its resolution or with practices that might be helpful in meeting the needs of the child.

What seems to be missing from this kind of orientation toward children with special needs is the relevance to education. Just as a physician could not be expected to recommend treatment based on a diagnostic label assigned to an unseen patient, neither can the educator be responsive to a label awarded to a child. Naming a disability sets into potential motion a vast set of generalizations, misconceptions, biases, and expectations that are unrelated to the individuality of the person. Reynolds and Balow have encouraged the establishment of alternative educational systems to meet the needs of such children. This strategy would remove the stigmatizing effect of personal categorization or classification and concentrate on identifying the functional capabilities of the child. Such an approach may be related to Lilly's (1970) proposal for the redefinition of exceptional children in general. Although not specifically directed to the education of children with physical disabilities, Lilly's proposal called attention to the concept of "exceptional situations within the school" (p. 48), rather than to exceptional children. Emphasizing school situations, and by extension, the learning interactions of teacher and child, is analogous to emphasizing the educational complexities of teaching and learning when the child is physically disabled, rather than the physical disability. Labeling a physically limiting disability provides no indication of the "exceptional situations within the school" for the child with the impairment. Indeed, it is assumed that an exceptional situation exists. This constitutes a basic premise for special education stagnation: an assumption. The assumption is that labels, pertaining to particular characteristics and consequences, can be applied to particular children regardless of the individuality of these children.

Two recent legislative actions provide great hope for children who have exceptional needs (including children with physical disabilities). One of these legislative provisions is contained in the administrative code cited previously and may seem benign on the surface; however it will, in fact, require a totally different conception of both regular and special education. Where, in the past, legislative statutes have referred to physically handicapped or mentally retarded pupils, this more recent identification and subsequent definition provide for an "individual with exceptional needs—a pupil whose education needs cannot be met by the regular classroom teacher with modification of the regular school program and who requires the benefit of special instruction and services" (California Administrative Code, 1977, Section 3301). This definition makes no assumption with regard to label, category, or classification. The implicit direction for implementation lies in the part of the definition that allows for participation of exceptional children in a regular school program when modification of this program is provided. This program modification has not been a part of previous legislative or administrative arrangements, but there is no suggestion that the special facilities, programs, and services required by individuals with exceptional needs will not be made available.

The Education for All Handicapped Children Act of 1975 (Public Law [PL] 94-142) has issued an even greater mandate for change in regard to children with exceptionalities. Within this law, two specifics are of particular note: (1) states will provide free and appropriate public education to *all* handicapped children regardless of the severity of their handicap and (2) in order for states to receive fiscal assistance, they must establish

> . . . procedures to assure that, to the maximum extent appropriate, handicapped children, including children in public or private institutions or other care facilities, are educated with children who are not handicapped, and that special classes, separate schooling, or other removal of handicapped children from the regular educational environment occurs only when the nature or severity of the handicap is such that education in regular classes with the use of supplementary aids and services cannot be achieved satisfactorily. (PL 94-142, Section 612, Part 5)

The Education for All Handicapped Children Act of 1975 will bring to the total field of special education opportunities that have not frequently been available in the past, including the interaction of children who are handicapped (according to the Act) and children who are normal in regular education settings. When this law becomes operational under the guidelines and timetables established for implementation, children with physical disabilities will be among those who will profit from its provisions.

Definitions of limitation based on self-concept or functioning levels

The previous discussion of disability has been based on the existence and use of various models, or professional descriptive techniques. Another approach to describing physical limitation involves a complex interaction of medical characteristics, the connotations that have been associated with the terminology, and the individual's self-concept. The terminology used in this book, as reflected in the title, emphasizes the presence of the individual with a descriptive modifier; *individuals with physical disabilities* seems preferable to *physically disabled individuals*. Although this preference may be considered by some as concerning only a choice of words and syntax, the implications are greater; it is still important to notice the choice of the word *disability* as opposed to other words that might have been used: *crippled, orthopedically handicapped, handicapped,* and so on. The terms disability, crippled, and handicapped do not appear in medical dictionaries in relation to their use as applied to the physical condition. Webster's (1970) definitions add some light to this word dilemma; according to this source, *cripple* refers to a person who is "lame or otherwise disabled in a way that prevents normal motion of the limbs or body"; for *disable,* the first choice of definitions is "to make unable, unfit or ineffective; cripple; incapacitate" for *handicap,* the third definition, and the one that seems to be most relevant for the discussion of physical limitations, is "something that hampers a person; disadvantage; hindrance." As is often the case, the dictionary does little to make a decision about which word to use, for best or universal meaning or understanding.

The literature on the psychology of disability is where the issue of word meaning and usage has been most frequently discussed. In this book *Stigma, Notes on the Management of Spoiled Identity,* Goffman (1963) suggests that there are three major types of stigma and that the first of these is "abominations of the body" (p. 4). This body alteration carries with it the following connotation: "By definition, of course, we believe the person with a stigma is not quite human. On this assumption we exercise varieties of discrimination, through which we effectively, if often unthinkingly, reduce his life chances" (p. 5).

It is this reduction of life chances that Wright (1960) refers to in her differentiation of the terms disability and handicap based on the limitations of physical functioning. Citing Hamilton (1950), Wright maintains that "a disability is a condition of impairment, physical or mental, having an objective aspect that can usually be described by a physician. . . . A handicap is the cumulative result of the obstacles which disability interposes between the individual and his maximum functional level" (p. 9). Here, then, we see the existence of both the objective and the subjective: the presence of observable, clinical phenomena and the relationship of these phenomena to the social, physical, and psychological life space of the individual; this life space is interpreted through firsthand interactions with the environment and through perceptions of the self and others.

Still another view concerning definitions and differentiation of labels is put forth by L'Abate and Curtis (1975). In discussing disability and handicap as meaningful terms, these authors introduce the term limitation as an additional consideration.

> Disability differs from impairment to the extent that it is the behavior pattern evolving from the limitations imposed upon an individual's capacities and levels of functioning by the impairment. Impairment is the actual physical defect, and disability is the behavior evolving from the impairment. Handi-

cap represents an individual's peculiar reactions to disability and impairment. It is the extent of an individual's subjective, negative use and interpretation of his disability and impairment. (p. 38)

To add to this ever-increasing lack of clarification of terms and their use and interpretation is the use of a specific medical diagnosis or term to identify a person and thus modify his individuality. Examples are as endless as the list of conditions to be diagnosed, but the following will be recognizable: the cerebral palsied (the CP), the muscular dystrophied or dystrophic (the MD), the amputee, and the arthritic.

At this point, one might ask, "What's the point?" "Does it make any difference?" As to the use of the terms, there is probably very little meaning that can be universal. A term used to describe an individual and where this adjective is placed in the description may be well understood by the user and misunderstood or rejected by others. It is this possibility of communication failure that makes terminology important. It is not the universality of terminology that governs our relations with people; rather, it is our efforts to understand or make clear whatever is being communicated that is important. The effort must be made to clarify what or who is referred to and in what context the reference is made.

Whether the term disability, handicap, or impairment is used, with or without an understood commonality of meaning, it must be put into context. Although there is no one accepted term that may be used to describe physical limitations, there is a need to put into perspective the base from which the terms are used. That base is the implied state of *normalcy*. If there are those who are disabled, by contrast there must be those who are abled (or able-bodied); if there are those who are handicapped, then there must be those who are nonhandicapped; and finally, if there are those who are impaired, then there must be those who are unimpaired. If there are those who are normal, must there be those who are abnormal? Even though *normal* may be difficult to define or communicate, every effort must be made to do so in a discussion of any of the terms used to describe the physical limitations of individuals. And, because *normal* may carry a variety of contingencies with it, it is clear that these contingencies need to be made explicit. The parameters of normalcy include, but are not limited to, time, place, and circumstance. What is normal functioning at one time may not be at other times; similarly, what is considered normal behavior in one place may be abnormal in another. Since disability implies deviation, that deviation must be used in content with a known standard: the normal model. This normal model, then, should be used as a reference and not as a model that all must strive to match and emulate.

The choice in this book is to use the term disability to refer to the objective, clinical occurrence of physical limitation and the term handicap to refer to the imposition of human and environmental circumstance on the individual with the disability. The normal condition from which the disability is recognized and identified consists of those physical attributes that fall within the range of activities and functionings of the majority of individuals. These attributes include ambulation, range of motion, coordination, muscle activities, fine and gross motor activities, and so on.

Effects of categorization

The effects of categorization take many forms, including the lack of individual identity, generalizations based on common labeling, and the forming of social reactions and attitudes. When a disability is considered as a whole, there are a variety of circumstances that may exert control over the reaction of the person who has physical limitations and the reactions of those who encounter the person with the disability. An attempt to relate to the disability is often a generalized response, rather than an individual response or a response to the person's individuality. The characteristics of the disability and the milieu in which the disability exists play a role in the response to and the reaction of persons with disabilities.

One of the more widely accepted formats for considering the effects of physical limitations on adjustment is that of the somatopsychological relationship (Wright, 1960). The somatopsychological approach considers the relationship of the variability of body characteristics on the behavioral functioning of the individual. As a result of research into the somatopsychological phenomena, Wright has stated that "somatic abnormality as a physical fact is not linked in a direct or simple way to psychological behavior. Heterogeneity of reaction to crippling is a necessary result" (p. 373). The following is an adaptation of Wright's generalizations concerning the somatopsychological relationship:

1. Persons with disabilities do not differ from others in regard to general adjustment. There are similar levels of overall adjustment and areas of overlap between the two groups.
2. A personality type associated with a particular disability cannot be established. There is no evidence to suggest that there is a cerebral palsy personality accompanying this particular set of physical deviations.
3. Although there is no evidence to suggest that a disability personality type exists, there are behaviors that are often associated with particular limitations. A cited example involves the difference in physical freedom between the person who is paraplegic as opposed to the person who is nondisabled. Where this physical behavioral difference may be considered almost as a given, the relationship between these differences to role adjustment is not clear.
4. "Physical disability has a profound effect on the person's life—" (p. 376). Even though there are no established group-related personality or adjustment characteristics that can be identified, it is nevertheless well established that adjustment strategies and conditions are quite individualized and personalized.
5. Public response to disability is only rarely at a negatively verbalized level.

This should not be too much of a surprise if we consider the implicit notion of the evils of talking out against the flag, motherhood, and the *downtrodden!* A lack of public negative verbalization may not be acceptable, but it is the unspoken response and the acts of nonverbal behavior that may give some clue as to the public's more general response to those with disabilities.

6. The reactions of parents to the child with a disability seem to be in the extreme as compared to their reactions to their normal children. These reactions range from overprotection to unrealistic expectations for a variety of behaviors.

7. There is a wide variety of attitudes held by persons who are disabled about their own disabilities. The variation in attitudes is dependent on the degree of disability, the type of personality before the onset of disability (if the disability was not congenital), value systems, and other influences that may add to self-directed attitudes toward the disability.

These very general responses to disability by groups and individuals with disabilities, and by parents and society at large, have as the foci of importance the highly individualized nature of disability, attitudes, adjustment, and personality. Response characteristics to disability depend on the age, sophistication, and experience of the individual or group investigated.

Attitudes and the forming of reactions or responses to labels may be influenced by other considerations, including the characteristics of those reporting their impressions of the disabled, as well as the characteristics of the disabled (Alessi and Anthony, 1969). The inability of physically limited persons to contribute to the work ethic, and hence their lack of productivity as perceived by others, may contribute to a negative interpretation of those with disabilities (Harasymia, Horne, and Lewis, 1976). Shears and Jensema (1969) have suggested the interaction of six disability characteristics contributing to the stereotypical reactions of others to those with disabilities:

1. Visibility of affliction
2. Interference in communication process
3. Social stigma
4. Reversibility prognosis
5. Extent of incapacity
6. Difficulties anomaly imposes on daily living routine (p. 96)

The effect of labels, or the ability of the nondisabled to interact with those with disabilities and vice versa, is of less value than the notion that we are, in fact, most concerned with the interaction of *people*. To be sure, there are influences that affect these interactions, but the prime consideration is the person-to-person interaction, not an adulated reference to generalized conditions.

The presence of persons with physical disabilities is not a phenomenon of recent history. It seems logical to suppose that even in the time before recorded history (life-styles) there were members of family groups, tribes, and so on, who were born with physical limitations or differences or who acquired physical disabilities that, in the sense of this book, became not only handicaps but deterrents to the life of the individual and/or group. The fact that the ancient Greeks were known to have abandoned their deformed children and the Biblical reference of a "man lame from his mother's womb" (Acts 3:12) may indicate the presence of cerebral palsy or other congenital "lameness" at these periods of history. Through the ages of western culture the disabled, crippled, and deformed have been variously subjected to ridicule, scorn, and death, and only recently to levels of protection and care. The asylums, prisons, and almshouses into which all of society's deviants were housed are light years away from the development of residential care facilities for children and adults with special needs and the provisions for education, training, and support services that are seen today. Through the raised voices of parents, individually and collectively, public demand for educational opportunity through special education, and most recently through an equal opportunity for education with their normal peers, has brought children with disabilities to the forefront with legal decisions establishing their rights as individuals.

DISABILITY POPULATION CHARACTERISTICS

Table 1 is presented to put into perspective the heterogeneity of the population making up the various physical disabilities found in the schools and to examine the other characteristics of a specific school population. The numbers and percentages reported in Table 1 represent two specific populations. The figures in the first column represent the numbers and percentages reported for specific disabilities identified in the public special day schools for children with physical disabilities in California. The figures in the second column represent numbers and percentages of disabilities from one specific school.

The figures in Table 1 are not a definitive statement regarding the distribution of disabilities in the California public schools, but they are notable for both consistency and inconsistency between the two columns in the reported types of disability. The best example of consistency in the reported figures is the similarity of size in the population figures for cerebral palsy. Although the state percentages show that more than half of the identified population of children with physical disabilities have cerebral palsy and the specific school population shows 40% of the school population with cerebral palsy, there is general consistency in these figures in that this disability type represents by far the majority of those occurring in the populations represented. Other similarities between the two columns are noted, including the percentages given for the incidence of Legg-Perthes disease and for muscular dystrophy. Dissimilar percentages are cited for the incidence of cardiac disorders, epilepsy, osteogenesis imperfecta, poliomyelitis, spina bifida, and the category of "others." To suggest that there is an explanation for the similarities and differences in the figures cited may be not only misleading, but also totally inaccurate. However, it is readily obvious that there is, in fact, a very heterogeneous population of children enrolled in the special schools for the physically disabled in

Table 1. Distribution of disabilities in California public schools for children with physical disabilities

Disability type	State Survey*		Special school survey†	
	N	Percentage of total	N	Percentage of total
Amputations	36	0.8	0	0
Amyotonia con-genita	45	1. +	0	0
Anomalies	115	2.6	2	2. +
Arthritis, rheuma-toid	41	0.9	0	0
Arthrogryposis	37	0.8	2	2. +
Cardiac disorders	103	2. +	0	0
Cerebral palsy	2,559	58. +	35	39.8
Epilepsy	83	1.8	4	4.5
Hemophilia	49	1. +	2	2. +
Legg-Perthes dis-ease	59	1. +	1	1. +
Muscular dystro-phy	287	6.5	7	7.9
Osteogenesis im-perfecta	28	0.6	2	2. +
Poliomyelitis	243	5.5	2	2. +
Spina bifida	185	4. +	9	10. +
Trauma	58	1. +	3	3. +
Others	465	10.5	19	21.6
	(Thirty-two identified different disabilities contributed to this category)		(Thirteen identified different disabilities contributed to this category)	
Total	4,393	100 (approximately)	88	100 (approximately)

*Adapted from Gore, B. E., and Outland, R. W. *Incidence report on types of handicaps found among children enrolled in special day schools for the orthopedically handicapped including the cerebral palsied in California (1965-66 school year)*. Sacramento: Department of Education, State of California, 1966.

†Adapted from the total enrollment figures for a special school for children with physical disabilities for the school year 1975-1976.

California. The presence or absence of differences in the reported figures may be due to such conditions as the availability of special schools and, hence, the identification of the occurrence of specific disabilities in a given population; the ability of a physician to make a definitive diagnosis; the mobility patterns of the families of the reported children; or differences in medical treatment and prevention capabilities, as might be seen in disability types such as cardiac disorders and poliomyelitis. Other considerations for disparity that might be taken into consideration for differences in reported incidence include the time periods of the reported surveys (1965-1966 and 1975-1976, a 10-year difference), possible differences in the severity of disability, and the prevailing administrative placement policies of the districts in which there are children with disabilities. There is, today, a movement toward the placement of children with various exceptionalities, including physical disabilities, in classes and schools with their normal peers. This placement process is dependent on the capabilities of the children; thus, this school placement procedure is limited to children whose disabilities would in most instances be described as "mild involvement." Since this is a relatively recent change in placement policy, there is likely to be reflected in more current population surveys figures that show either (1) an overall lower absolute or proportionate decrease in incidence based on general population growth or (2) decrease in incidence for certain of the disabilities represented, with fewer children cited as having "mild" levels of disability.

Although the figures presented in Table 1 may be of interest to the academician, statistician, or researcher, they may hold little more than passing significance for the person who might be contemplating entrance into the field of teaching children with physical disabilities or for the professional already in the field. Of more importance than a comparison of incidence figures, or even the presence or absence of a specific disability, is the question of what a teacher or administrator might expect to find in terms of the disabilities, ages, sex distribution, and functioning levels of children in a given special school. These characteristics are the ones that will be important to the teacher and/or administrator because they represent the actual children (although not their actual behaviors).

To provide a more realistic picture of what might be expected in regard to population characteristics of a special school for children with physical disabilities, the data from the second column of Table 1 are expanded in Table 2. Table 2 represents the characteristics of a total school population on several dimensions: (1) specific classes by grade level identification, (2) disability type for each class member in each class, (3) sex of each class member, (4) intelligence quotient (IQ) score of each class member based on the results of an individually administered intelligence test, and (5) severity of disability. Three degrees or levels of involvement of the children in each of the eight reported classes are given. These school-defined levels are "mild" (a child who is ambulatory, has little or no speech involvement, and who is able to care for himself/herself); "moderate" (a child who is ambulatory but who uses aids, has some speech involvement, and requires some help in personal care); and "severe" (a child who is wheelchair bound, has considerable speech involvement, and requires a significant amount of help in personal care). It is readily apparent that these levels of disability may be arbitrary and in many respects of a generalized nature; they are used here only as broad categories of involvement.

The distribution of characteristics of children in Table 2 have several interest-

Table 2. Characteristics of children enrolled in an elementary school for the physically disabled

Class	Disability	Sex	IQ	Severity
Preschool; chronological ages (CA): 3-5 approximately	Cerebral palsy	F	31	Severe
	Cerebral palsy	F	97	Mild
	Cerebral palsy	F	35	Severe
	Cerebral palsy	F	100	Moderate
	Cerebral palsy	M	90	Mild
	Cerebral palsy	M	45	Mild
	Cerebral palsy	M	35	Moderate
	Hemophilia	M	100	Mild
	Muscle weakness	M	63	Moderate
	Spina bifida	F	80	Moderate
	Spina bifida	F	88	Moderate
Preschool-kindergarten; CA: 5-6 approximately	Cerebral palsy	M	71	Moderate
	Cerebral palsy	F	50	Moderate
	Muscle weakness	M	87	Mild
	Spina bifida	M	63	Severe
	Post-meningitis	F	59	Moderate
	Epilepsy	M	*	Mild
	Epilepsy	F	44	Mild
	Severe speech disorder†	F	84	Mild
Kindergarten; CA: 5-6 approximately	Cerebral palsy	M	108	Moderate
	Cerebral palsy	F	147	Moderate
	Cerebral palsy	M	136	Moderate
	Cerebral palsy	F	124	Moderate
	Hemophilia	M	108	Mild
	Spina bifida	M	102	Mild
	Tracheotomy	F	126	Mild
	Spina bifida	M	149	Mild
	Post-head trauma	M	111	Moderate
	Post-polio	F	128	Moderate
	Muscular dystrophy	M	114	Moderate
First grade; CA: 6-7 approximately	Cerebral palsy	F	77	Moderate
	Cerebral palsy	F	100	Moderate
	Cerebral palsy	M	67	Moderate
	Epilepsy (with cerebral palsy)	M	79	Moderate
	Arthrogryposis	F	57	Moderate
	Spina bifida	F	89	Mild
	Post-burn	F	110	Mild
	Muscular dystrophy	M	90	Mild
	Achondroplasia/macrocephaly	M	59	Mild
	Spina bifida	F	94	Moderate
	Legg-Perthes disease	F	100	Moderate

*Unable to determine at testing.   *Continued.*
†Children with severe speech disorders may be enrolled in this school in order to receive intensive speech/language therapy.

Table 2. Characteristics of children enrolled in an elementary school for the physically disabled—cont'd

Class	Disability	Sex	IQ	Severity
Second-third grade; CA: 8-9 approximately	Cerebral palsy	M	135	Moderate
	Cerebral palsy	M	58	Mild
	Cerebral palsy	F	95	Severe
	Cerebral palsy	M	55	Mild
	Arthrogryposis	M	79	Severe
	Muscular dystrophy	M	61	Severe
	Muscular dystrophy	M	118	Moderate
	Post-polio	M	109	Moderate
	Bone tumors	F	83	Mild
	Severe speech disorder*	M	93	Mild
Intermediate (identified learning disabilities in addition to physical disabilities); CA: 8-15 approximately	Cerebral palsy	M	47	Severe
	Cerebral palsy	F	64	Moderate
	Cerebral palsy	M	77	Mild
	Cerebral palsy	F	64	Severe
	Cerebral palsy	F	55	Moderate
	Cerebral palsy	M	61	Moderate
	Muscular dystrophy	M	66	Moderate
	Hydrocephally	F	41	Moderate
	Post-head trauma	F	73	Severe
	Severe speech disorder*	F	67	Mild
Fourth-fifth grade; CA: 10-12 approximately	Cerebral palsy	F	116	Moderate
	Cerebral palsy	F	91	Mild
	Cerebral palsy	F	106	Severe
	Cerebral palsy	F	94	Moderate
	Upper-extremity birth anomalies	M	87	Mild
	Peripheral nerve disease	M	123	Mild
	Multiple congenital anomalies	F	90	Mild
	Osteogenesis imperfecta	M	125	Moderate
	Osteogenesis imperfecta	M	105	Mild
	Muscular dystrophy	M	91	Moderate
	Hurler's syndrome	F	77	Moderate
	Bone tumors	M	94	Mild
	Werdnig-Hoffman disease	F	107	Severe
Sixth-eighth grade; CA: 12-15 approximately	Cerebral palsy	M	97	Moderate
	Cerebral palsy	M	68	Moderate
	Cerebral palsy	F	100	Moderate
	Cerebral palsy	F	64	Mild
	Cerebral palsy	F	78	Moderate
	Spina bifida	F	96	Moderate
	Spina bifida	F	86	Moderate
	Hydrocephally	F	83	Mild
	Polymyositis	M	99	Moderate
	Muscular dystrophy	M	89	Severe
	Post-head trauma	M	85	Severe
	Prader-Willi syndrome	F	66	Moderate
	Post-meningitis	M	74	Moderate
	Epilepsy	M	76	Mild

ing features. It is taken for granted that these population characteristics are representative of the school from which they were drawn and not of the total population of children with physical disabilities. The school used to supply the figures in Table 2 is relatively small and contains only the elementary grades. There is some suggestion that population characteristics change in the high school. This may be accounted for, in part, by the enrollment of persons in high schools for the disabled who have more severe involvement and by the enrollment of those with a lesser degree of involvement in integrated classes in regular high schools or in special classes on regular school campuses.

A careful look at the list of disabilities occuring in the school population represented in Table 2 shows that there are several disabilities that are not found and yet might be expected within a population of children with disabilities in a special education facility: cardiac disabilities, arthritis, cystic fibrosis, amputations, and others. However, the list is presented as an exact representation of a given school for a given school year. The school from which this survey was made has recently changed in its disability representation because of an influx of approximately 15 children with varying degrees of involvement from poliomyelitis. These children, who are Vietnamese refugees, may be found at all grade levels throughout the school and have thus caused a dramatic increase in the incidence of post-polio disabilities in that population.

Other characteristics of the population in Table 2 are worth noting: (1) there is an almost even split between the sexes for the total number of disabilities in the school—45 boys and 43 girls—and (2) distribution of levels of involvement for the school population as a whole indicates that there are more who need some help for their physical care than there are those who are able to care for themselves—31 children have mild levels of involvement, 44 have moderate levels and 13 have severe levels.

The characteristic of the school population that may have the most significance for the classroom teacher is the distribution of IQ scores for the children. Although it is accepted that a given score on an IQ test does not necessarily reflect the academic behavior of the child, such scores may provide some insight into the measured levels of intellectual functioning. Even though questions are raised about the methods of measuring intelligence for children who may have difficulty with the peculiarities of test administration and not with the test content itself, the reported IQ figures do offer some indication of the presence of multiple disabilities, physical and mental.

Fig. 1-1 shows the distribution of intelligence for the school population that was surveyed. It is easily seen that there is a very negatively skewed distribution of IQ scores with the highest frequency occurring at the lower end. It should be reemphasized that the figures presented are not a definitive study and in no way are meant to imply large-sample characteristics. The teacher may find, however, this data to be more interesting than studies supplying characteristics of large numbers of children. The distribution of IQ scores here is not unlike those reported in a

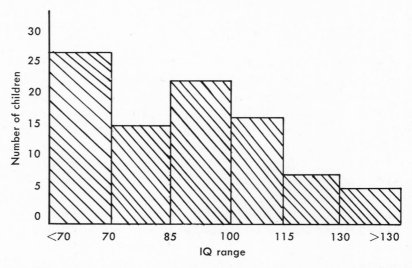

Fig. 1-1. Intelligence distribution of students enrolled in an elementary school for physically disabled children.

summary of research on IQ scores in populations of children with cerebral palsy (Connor, Rusalem, and Cruickshank, 1971); when considering such figures, however, one must also take into account the overall functioning of an individual child or group of children. The problems inherent in tests, the capability of children to manipulate test materials, and the environmental factors that may have limited the child from active exploration, tend to make any group data somewhat meaningless.

The greatest single action that might be taken, then would be for one to strip away the facts and figures from any reported population and be prepared to interact with the human behavioral characteristics of individuals. As suggested by Perls in *The Gestalt Prayer,* it is neither simplistic nor idealistic to consider such interactions. The implications are staggering and demand attention to all the characteristics of Perls's *you* and *I.*

The Gestalt Prayer*

I do my thing, and you do your thing.
I am not in this world to live up to your expectations
And you are not in this world to live up to mine.
You are you and I am I,
And if by chance we find each other, it's beautiful.
If not, it can't be helped.*

THE CHANGING POPULATION

If there is a truism about physical disabilities and their associated features, characteristics, services, and so on, it is that change is continual. There are fewer children with postpolio involvement in the special schools and classes today than there were several years ago; there are more children who have multiple disabilities and severe levels of involvement in special classes and schools today; there are more services available to those with disabilities and their families today than ever before; there is a growing public awareness and concern about the needs, rights, and demands of those with disabilities; and parenthetically, there is a greater involvement by those with disabilities in expressing their needs and in voicing their rights and demands. There have been parents who have demanded educational and treatment services for their special children; there have been advances made in the professions that treat and serve those with disabilities; there have been wars that have brought societal attention to the victims who have returned with a loss of physical *wholeness* to the society from which they left physically *whole*; and there have been, and continue to be, legal decisions and legislative mandates requiring change from what once was to what is now expected and ought to be.

It has been said that there has not really been a civil rights movement or a revolution for the rights of women; rather, there has been an evolution of these rights and their expression. This evolutionary function of equal rights has been extended to those with disabilities. Perhaps most notable among the efforts to establish change for those with disabilities has been the enunciation of the direction toward which change should be aimed. This directionality has been expressed through documents or statements declaring the rights and needs that have been denied or at least not seriously attributed to those with disabilities. Two such statements are presented here for consideration.

A BILL OF RIGHTS FOR THE DISABLED*

Whereas, the disabled in the United States, constituting a large minority with a personality of need and a unity of purpose, seek only to obtain for themselves what all Americans believe to be their birthright—life, liberty and the pursuit of happiness; and

Whereas, impediments and roadblocks of every nature are to be found at every bend, effectively preventing the fulfillment of life's promise for a large proportion of the disabled; and

Whereas, the American people, largely through lack of knowledge and misinformation have not as yet recognized the disabled as fellow human beings

---

* From Abramson, S., and Kutner, B. A bill of rights for the disabled. *Archives of Physical Medicine and Rehabilitation*, 1972, 53, 99-100.

with a handicap to which all should make some accomodation, and who deserve equal opportunity as citizens; and

Whereas, the Congress of the United States and the legislatures of the various cities, counties and municipalities have not as yet, by legal means, made it possible for the disabled person to attain equal access to those benefits of life enjoyed by the able bodied, be it resolved:

Health—1

That all disabled persons be afforded the opportunity for full and comprehensive diagnostic, therapeutic, rehabilitative and follow-up services in the nation's hospitals, clinics and rehabilitation centers without regard to race, religion, economic status, ethnic origin, sex, age, or social condition.

Health—2

That all disabled persons requiring same be given and trained to use such orthotic, prosthetic or adaptive devices that will enable them to become more mobile and to live more comfortably.

Education—3

That all disabled persons be given every opportunity for formal education to the level of which they are capable and to the degree to which they aspire.

Employment—4

That all disabled persons, to the extent necessary, have the opportunity to receive special training commensurate with the residual abilities in those aspects of life in which they are handicapped, so that they may achieve the potential for entry into the labor market in competitive employment.

Employment—5

That all employable disabled persons, like other minorities, be covered by equal opportunity legislation so that equal productivity, potential and actual, receives equal consideration in terms of jobs, promotions, salaries, workloads and fringe benefits.

Employment—6

That those disabled persons who because of the severity of their handicaps are deemed unable to enter the normal labor market, be given the opportunity for special training and placement in limited work situations including sheltered workshops, home-base employment and other protected job situations.

Employment—7

That a nationwide network of tax-supported sheltered workshops be created to offer limited work opportunities for all those severely disabled persons unable to enter the competitive labor market.

Housing—8

That nationwide and local programs of special housing for the disabled be established to permit them an opportunity to live in dignity and reasonable comfort.

Architectural barriers—9

That federal, state and local legislatures pass laws requiring the elimination of architectural barriers to buildings, recreational, cultural and social facilities and public places. Such legislation should include architectural standards for all new construction.

Architectural barriers—10

That federal, state and local legislation be passed establishing standards and a reasonable time for modification of existing sidewalks, buildings and structures for the comfortable use of the handicapped.

Transportation—11

That every community, county or other legally constituted authority establish programs and standards for the creation of special transportation for the disabled including modification of existing mass transportation systems and the development of new specially designed demand-schedule transportation facilities.

Income maintenance—12

That every disabled person who because of the nature of his handicap is unable to be self-supporting, be given a guaranteed minimum income not below established federal standards adequate to live in reasonable comfort and in dignity.

Institutional care—13

That federal, state and local laws be enacted for the benefit of the disabled confined to any form of institution, setting minimum standards of housing, conveniences, comfort, staff and services.

Civil rights—14

That civil rights legislation, national and local, be amended to include disability as one of the categories against which discrimination is unlawful.

Training—15

That federal and state tax-supported programs of training be established to prepare professional and nonprofessional personnel for work with the handicapped in the fields of health, education, recreation and welfare.

Research—16

That federal legislation be enacted expanding existing and developing new programs of research and demonstration, by grant and contract, in both basic and applied fields, dealing with the problems of disabling conditions and the disabled.

Be it further resolved that these rights, being urgent and critical to the well-being of the disabled population of the United States, be given the high priority they justly deserve in the hearts, minds, and programs of our nation's leaders.

A Bicentennial Declaration of Human Rights For Handicapped Persons*

When in the Course of human events, it becomes necessary for a people to dissolve the bonds which have constrained them, and to assume among the powers of the earth the separate and equal station to which the Laws of Nature and Nature's God entitle them, a decent respect to the opinions of human kind requires that they should declare the causes which impel them to the declaration.

We hold these truths to be self-evident, that all people are created equal, that they are endowed by their Creator with certain unalienable rights, that among these are Life, Liberty and the pursuit of Happiness.

We further declare that for the physically handicapped, the paramount right is to be a person made whole by exercising human potentialities, most notably:

The right to citizenship
No person shall be denied this right by inaccessible buildings or polling places. For each person it shall be made possible to vote, and to enter freely and do business independently in public buildings such as the courts, social service and employment offices, city halls, and county buildings.

The right to educate oneself
No physically handicapped person shall be denied equal opportunity to utilize educational institutions, libraries, museums, or other means of pursuing knowledge by reason of architectural, traditional, or attitudinal barriers.

The right to an occupation or profession
No person shall be denied the right to enter any occupation or profession solely for reasons of disability, provided he or she can perform the duties of the occupation creditably.

The right to maintain health and physical wellbeing
Medical facilities shall provide equal access to all persons regardless of physical or other disabilities; moreover, public facilities shall be made generally available, identifiable, and accessible to handicapped persons including food service, restrooms, and places to have a drink of water or to rest when tired.

The right to recreation
No persons shall be denied access by reason of physical handicap to auditoriums, theaters, sports facilities, public parks and monuments, woodlands,

*From Westie, C. M. *A bicentennial declaration of human rights for handicapped persons.* Mt. Pleasant: Central Michigan University, Office of Career Development for Handicapped Persons, 1976.

rivers, lakes or other recreational or entertainment facilities open to the general public.

The right to independent living

Handicapped persons shall not be denied accomodations in houses, apartments, hotels, dormitories, or barracks open to other persons, and shall be free to live with other persons of their choice.

The right to safe and independent travel

No citizen, government regulatory agency, or public carrier shall prevent handicapped persons from equal access to any mode of transportation. Public agencies shall do all in their power to facilitate the safe movement of physically handicapped persons.

The right to love

No citizen, agency, or any legislative, executive, or judicial branch of government shall deny to handicapped persons the relationships of friendship, love, and marriage through any means not applicable to all other persons.

The right to worship

Handicapped persons shall be afforded the means to enter places of worship independently and the right to attend public worship services.

The right to live and die with dignity

No person shall be denied the right to live with dignity, and, when finding life no longer bearable, to die with dignity, within the legal requirements of the state in which he or she lives.

We therefore declare, on the occasion of the two-hundredth birthday of our beloved country, that physically handicapped people are and of a right ought to be free and independent, and that such persons have the power to live as independent and full human beings. We who subscribe to this declaration shall do all things in our power to secure these rights, and for the support of this declaration, we mutually pledge to each other our lives, our fortunes, and our sacred honor.

The reader of these two statements should not have difficulty imagining what King George III of England must have felt while reading that pretentious little document from the colonies when they declared their independence from Great Britain. Rather than taxation without representation, the cause today is existence without participation. This participation in the social, economic, personal, and political life-styles of the normal majority have been implicitly and explicitly denied to those with disabilities. Since the enumeration of these rights and demands, there have been efforts to alleviate at least some of these discriminatory practices through both federal legislation and executive order. These actions have included the requirements of accessibility to buildings that used federal financing in their construction; affirmative action in employment practices (including provisions for those with disabilities); and a section of the Vietnam Era Veterans Readjustment Assistance Act of 1974, which also provides for affirmative action in employment practices for those veterans who were disabled during service in the Vietnam war era.

Declarations and statements of rights, the passing of legislation, and the issuing of executive orders are, however, not sufficient to compensate for the inherent lack of equality of those with disabilities. This lack of equality is a fact that is easily forgotten, ignored, or even rejected by many; and in that respect it will continue to be a problem of great magnitude. Perhaps the greater problem, though, is the nature of the human condition that seems to promote the exclusion of the perceived abnormal. It is this rejection—this perception of abnormality—and the human characteristic of comparing and measuring individuals against each other that must be changed if there is ever to be a full and mutual concordance of life's benefits.

SUMMARY

This chapter has established the base for the terminology used throughout the book; *disability* is presented as the term of choice to connote the objective characteristic of a physical limitation or the medical diagnosis used to describe a set of symptoms. The importance lies not with selection of disability as a term, however, but with the placement of that word in relation to the person for whom it is an appropriate descriptor. The emphasis is on the *person* with a disability, not on a disabled person.

The size of the population is briefly discussed in terms of what one might find in a special school for children with physical disabilities. This population characteristic is more meaningful than a set of national statistics of the frequency of incidence for a group of disabilities. Of significance is the changing nature of the population of children with disabilities and the patterns of school placement as a result of PL 94-142, the Education for All Handicapped Children Act of 1975.

Bills of rights, written by and for those with disabilities, are becoming documents of action as persons with disabilities become more a part of, rather than apart from, the majority of the population as represented by the able-bodied. An abridgement of rights can no longer be tolerated by the many against the few.

REFERENCES

Abramson, S., and Kutner, B. A bill of rights for the disabled. *Archives of Physical Medicine and Rehabilitation*, 1972, *53*, 99-100.

Alessi, D. F., and Anthony, W. A. The uniformity of children's attitudes toward physical disabilities. *Exceptional Children*, 1969, *35*, 543-545.

California Administrative Code. *Title 5, Califor-*

nia Administrative Code. Sacramento: Office of Administrative Hearings, Department of General Services, State of California, 1977.

California Education Code. *California Education Code, 1976.* Sacramento: Department of General Services, State of California, 1976.

Connor, F. P., Rusalem, H., and Cruickshank, W. M. Psychological considerations with crippled children. In W. M. Cruickshank (Ed.), *Psychology of exceptional children and youth* (3rd ed). Englewood Cliffs, N.J.: Prentice-Hall, Inc., 1971.

Goffman, E. *Stigma, notes on the management of spoiled identity.* Englewood Cliffs, N.J.: Prentice-Hall, Inc., 1963.

Gore, B. E., and Outland, R. W. *Incidence report on types of handicaps found among children enrolled in special day schools for the orthopedically handicapped including the cerebral palsied in California (1965-66 school year).* Sacramento: Department of Education, State of California, 1966.

Hamilton, K. W. Counseling the handicapped in the rehabilitation process. New York: Ronald Press, 1950. Cited in B. A. Wright, *Physical disability—a psychological approach.* New York: Harper & Row, Publishers, Inc., 1960, p. 17.

Harasymia, S. J., Horne, M. D., and Lewis, S. C. A longitudinal study of disability group acceptance. *Rehabilitation Literature,* 1976, 37, 98-102.

L'Abate, L. and Curtis, L. T. *Teaching the exceptional child.* Philadelphia: W. B. Saunders Co., 1975.

Lilly, M. S. Special education: a teapot in a tempest. *Exceptional Children,* 1970, 37, 43-49.

Perls, F. *Gestalt therapy verbatim.* Lafayette, Calif.: Real People Press, 1969.

PL 94-142. *Education for All Handicapped Children Act of 1975.*

Reynolds, M. C., and Balow, B. Categories and variables in special education. *Exceptional Children,* 1972, 38, 357-366.

Shears, L. M., and Jensema, C. J. Social acceptability of anomalous persons. *Exceptional Children,* 1969, 36, 91-96.

Webster's new world dictionary of the American language (2nd college ed.). New York: World Publishing, 1970.

Westie, C. M. *A bicentennial declaration of human rights for handicapped persons.* Mt. Pleasant: Central Michigan University, Office of Career Development for Handicapped Persons, 1976.

Wright, B. A. *Physical disability—a psychological approach.* New York: Harper & Row, Publishers, Inc., 1960.

2 Cerebral palsy

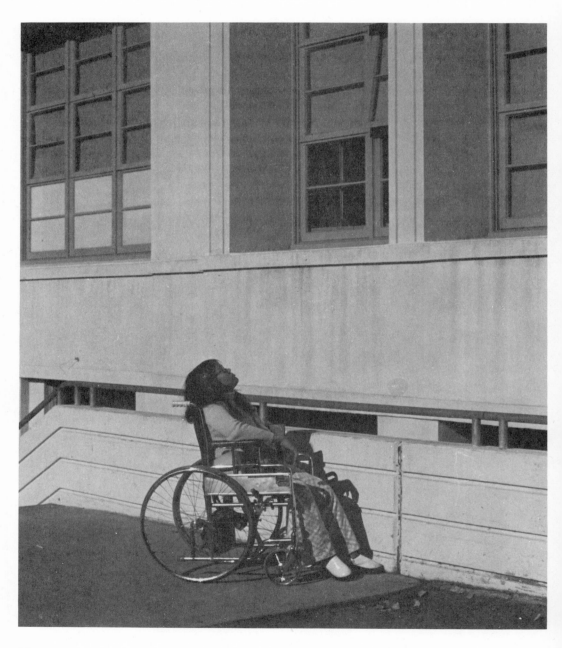

NEUROLOGICAL IMPAIRMENT

Because cerebral palsy as a physical disability is the result of damage or injury to the brain, it is best to consider the various components of neurological (brain) impairment. As might be expected, there is a significant question that arises with regard to terminology. The specificity of the terms used by professionals between and within specialities has led to considerable misunderstanding and lack of clear communication. Neurological impairment is operationally defined here as abnormal performance arising out of dysfunction of a specific part of the central nervous system: the brain. Although this definition appears to be broad in scope, it is within this context that much miscommunication, or even failure in communication, occurs and the need for clarification arises. Looking at the definition first and then trying to find terminology to match the meaning is an exercise that will add to the frustration often felt by those who assume that there is a universal understanding of what is being said. For example, the definition of neurological impairment provided above might be equally appropriate for each of the following conditions, labels, or terms: neurological damage, brain damage, central nervous system damage, central nervous system impairment, minimal brain damage, minimal brain dysfunction, and other signs, symptoms, or conditions of deficiency or deficit. Different individuals may well use the same terminology to express problems related to physical motor functioning, intellectual and/or learning functioning, speech and/or language functioning, behavioral functioning, or combinations of these and others.

Underlying this terminology problem is a commonality that should be apparent when one considers the base structure and feature of all the foregoing: the brain. Of all that is known about the brain, there is still an amount to be learned that is some unknown mathematical factor beyond that which is already acknowledged. This nervous tissue mass consists of hemispheres, lobes, fissures, ventricles, and other interrelated parts, such as the medulla oblongata, the pons, the cerebrum, and the cerebellum. These features provide direction to all of the body's functions and behaviors. Damage to a part or parts of the brain results in impairment of function and performance of the body system that is controlled by the affected part(s). Fig. 2-1 diagrammatically represents the consequences of damage to the brain (the nature of the damage or its specific location are not considered).

The six major areas of disturbance or dysfunction as a result of injury to the brain are related to specific sites of damage: these sites and related areas of functioning include physical activity (impaired motor function), intellectual ability (mental retardation), behavioral consequences (lack of attention or inhibition control, for example) state of consciousness (epilepsy and associated seizure activity), sensory functioning (impaired acuity and perception), and communication involvement (impaired language processing and speech production). It is little wonder, then, that when the term *brain damage* is used by individuals of the same or different profession, the likelihood for miscommunication occurs, even if the conditions for the interchange are set and known.

DEFINITIONS

At this point, the reader should feel very little surprise to learn that the condition known as cerebral palsy does not have a universally accepted definition. A review of the vast amount of literature that has been written in both the medical and educational professions reveals that there are practically no two definitions the same, unless one author uses a definition given by another. Several of the definitions that have been used are presented here so that the reader may compare them and perhaps select one for personal use:

> Any abnormal alteration of movement or motor function arising from defect, injury, or disease of the nervous tissues contained in the cranial cavity. (Cardwell, 1956, p. 4)

> Cerebral palsy is a manifestation or group of manifestations of impaired neurologic function due to aberrant structure, growth, or development of the central nervous system. (Denhoff and Robinault, 1960, p. 1)

> Cerebral palsy is not a single disease entity, but comprises a group of syndromes with the common denominator of a chronic motor disability due to involvement of the motor control centers in the brain. (Perlstein and Hood, 1964, p. 850)

> . . . any disorder that is characterized by a non-progressive motor abnormality, with or without sensory impairment and/or mental retardation, due to injury or disease of the brain that is manifested before the fifth birthday. (Malamud, Itabashi, and Castor, 1964, p. 271)

> Cerebral palsy is a general term used to designate any paralysis, weakness, incoordination, or functional deviation of the motor system resulting from an intracranial lesion. (Keats, 1965, p. 6)

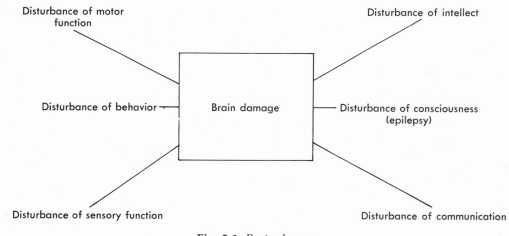

Fig. 2-1. Brain damage.

> ... refers to a static motor disorder of the brain, due to in utero factors, events that may occur at birth or in the neonatal period (congenital cerebral palsy) or in the early developmental years (acquired cerebral palsy). (Scherzer, 1974, p. 194)

The definitions cited above have few commonalities that might be useful in developing a clear understanding of the oft-used term cerebral palsy. Two of these definitions use the terms *nervous tissue* or *central nervous system,* whereas others variously use the word *brain* to describe the location of the damage. Some of the definitions include results of the brain damage or specific areas of the brain that are damaged; others include the causes of brain damage or the time during which the damage should occur for a diagnosis of cerebral palsy to be made. Although a distinction is made or implied between congenital cerebral palsy (the condition associated with the birth or prebirth period) and acquired cerebral palsy (the condition occurring after the birth period) there is little clarification regarding the time period that might be included for the acquired form of cerebral palsy. The definitions cited by Cardwell; Denhoff and Robinault; Perlstein and Hood; and Keats do not identify an age reference, whereas Malamud and others use the fifth birthday and Scherzer gives "the early developmental years" as the time period included for acquired cerebral palsy.

If it is important to have a definition of cerebral palsy, an arbitrary selection can be made from the many that have been offered. A combination of bits and pieces from several sources, Table 3 is an attempt to identify what others have said cerebral palsy *is* or *is not*.

Because cerebral palsy is a complexity of characteristics, causes, and other associated clinical descriptions, it is necessary for one to put cerebral palsy into perspective. Cerebral palsy as a term may serve as a hub from which spokes of association may be drawn (Fig. 2-2). These spokes are examined in the rest of this chapter, beginning with the motor component (one method of classification) and moving counterclockwise.

Table 3. Cerebral palsy

Is	Is not
Related to damage to motor control areas of the brain	A disease
Nonprogressive	Curable
Static	Terminal
A group of syndromes	Often a single syndrome entity
Impaired neurological function	
Manifested by motor and postural disorders	
A neuromotor aspect of brain damage	
Amenable to treatment	

Fig. 2-2. Cerebral palsy and associated characteristics.

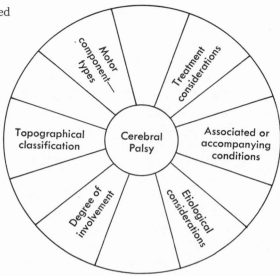

CLASSIFICATION
Motor types

In a classification scheme developed by Minear (1956) and adopted by the American Academy for Cerebral Palsy, the motor component aspect of cerebral palsy is given precedence over other forms of classification. Within the motor component, six types of cerebral palsy have emerged: spasticity, athetosis, ataxia, rigidity, tremor, and mixed.

Spasticity. The spastic form of cerebral palsy is the most common type; its reported percentage of the total number of cases of cerebral palsy occurring in a population ranges from 48.4% for the 1965-1966 California survey (Gore and Outland, 1966) to 81.2% (Morris, 1973). Denhoff (1976) has reported an incidence of 50% to 60% for spasticity, which might be taken as a compromise average of the many incidence figures that have been reported.

The physical characteristics found in the individual with spastic-type cerebral palsy include "a tendency toward greater involvement and contractures [a fixed condition of muscles] affecting the antigravity muscles" (Minear, 1956, pp. 845-846). When stretched passively or actively, the antigravity muscles, such as the biceps (gravity muscles are triceps), tend to contract, resulting in tense, difficult, and often inaccurate, though voluntary, movement. Involvement in the upper extremities may include varying degrees of flexion of the arms and fingers, depending on the severity of the spasticity. When the lower extremities are involved, there may be a "scissoring" movement of the legs, caused by muscle contraction, which "draws the legs together and often rotates them inward at the hip joint" (Cardwell, 1956, p. 85). There may also be a toe-walking–type gait, which results from an inwardly rotated foot and from a contraction of the calf muscles causing elevation of the foot on the toes.

Not all of the physical characteristics may be present at any given time in the individual. Symptoms may elude detection in very young children because of the normal lack of sophistication of muscle activity. The abnormal muscle activity, tone, and positioning of the child with spastic-type cerebral palsy may become evident when the child fails to reach normal milestones in physical development—when the child fails to exercise the natural infant perogative of muscle exploration, strengthening, and development for physical independence.

Athetosis. The athetotic form of cerebral palsy accounts for the second largest group of cerebral palsy types. The incidence figures range from 11.5% (reported by Morris) to 13.6% percent (reported by Gore and Outland). Denhoff's figures, 20% to 25%, include the athetosic type as well as the more infrequently occurring rigid and tremor types. As with the figures for the spastic type, the range is considerable for the athetosic type; hence, incidence figures between study groups will nearly always lack uniformity because of population variation.

According to Minear, several forms of athetosis are recognized by the majority of the members of the American Academy for Cerebral Palsy. These forms include tension, nontension, dystonia, and tremor. A general description of the characteristic physical symptoms of athetosis include involuntary muscle activity consisting of a writhing, irregular constant motion. The activity tends to be located in the proximal parts of the extremities and face; there is extension and spread of the fingers, and the head is drawn back with the mouth open and the tongue protruding (Cardwell, 1956). The uncontrolled movements are less noticeable when the individual is at rest and disappear during sleep. However, when the individual is under stress or emotional tension, the involuntary motions may become more pronounced.

The tension and nontension forms of athetosis are not constant in their presence and may "mask other types of athetosis" (Minear, 1956, p. 846). The muscle tension or lack of it in the two respective forms of athetosis are characteristically present in the very young infant and are used only temporarily as classifications (Denhoff and Robinault, 1960). Bartram (1969) has stated that it is "only during the second year . . . [that] the fine wandering movement of the fingers, hands and feet become evident and develop into the typical pattern of athetosis" (p. 1312).

The dystonic form of athetosis, which may involve the neck, trunk, arms, and legs, may result in distorted positions for a few seconds or minutes, followed by a change in the position pattern (Minear, 1956). This type of uncontrolled motion is in contrast to the constancy of motion most frequently seen in athetosis.

The tremor form of athetosis, though not a true tremor (Denhoff and Robinault, 1960), is characterized by "an irregular and uneven type of involuntary contraction and relaxation which involves flexor and extensor, and abduction and adduction mechanisms" (Minear, 1956, p. 846).

Ataxia, rigidity, and tremor. Three other types of cerebral palsy include ataxia, rigidity, and tremor. These forms are combined for discussion not because of their similarity of characteristics but because of their lack of frequency of occurrence in the total cerebral palsy population. Morris reported in his study population that, after the spastic and athetotic forms of cerebral palsy were considered, the remaining types accounted for only 7.3%. These forms of cerebral palsy are infrequently seen in the classroom and may be seen in association with other forms, such as athetosis or spasticity.

The ataxic form of cerebral palsy is characterized by a lack of coordination and sense of balance. This disturbance of equilibrium appears most conspicuously in attempts at walking wherein the individual may appear to defy the laws of gravity; frequent falls mark the difficulty with which this activity occurs. Bleck (1975) has described children with ataxia and their characteristic walking pattern "as if they were sailors on a rolling ship at sea—feet apart and weaving of the trunk with arms akimbo to balance" (p. 43).

Rigidity is an infrequently occuring form of cerebral palsy and may be a severe form of the spastic type (Bleck, 1975). The rigid type of cerebral palsy is often associated with the terms *lead pipe* type or *cogwheel* type, depending on the specificity of the characteristic present in the child. The leadpipe type of rigidity refers to the constant resistance to movement and has been compared to the stiffness of a leadpipe; the cogwheel type shares the resistance to movement of the leadpipe type, but the resistance lacks constancy; hence it may appear more intense at one time and less at others. The overall characteristic of the rigid type of cerebral palsy is the presence of high levels of muscle tone (hypertonicity) and the lack of voluntary motion.

The tremor form of cerebral palsy is characterized by the presence of involuntary motion. This motion may vary in its constancy and pattern. Direction and purpose of movement toward a motor goal is more successful than in either the spastic or athetotic form (Cardwell, 1956). The overall appearance of the tremor is that of a shaking or trembling of the limb.

Mixed types. Although not a *pure* form of cerebral palsy, this combination of types should be considered. The importance in this consideration is particularly relevant to the functioning of the child who may show a combined form of cerebral palsy. It is not infrequent that one finds a child with cerebral palsy in the classroom who may demonstrate both the tenseness of movement of the spastic type and the lack of control associated with the athetotic type. This multiple interference of movement produces an increased lack of motor volition or planning. Although one of the major forms may be more prominent than another in the mixed type, there seems to be a growing recognition that this "nontype" is occurring with more frequency than had been previously noted. The California data of 1965-1966 (Gore and Outland, 1966,) indicates that the mixed type accounted for only 2.7% of the population, whereas a more recent statement of occurrence indicates an incidence of 15% to 40% (Denhoff, 1976). As in other population studies, a fluctuation in numbers may be expected in the contributions of individuals for different population studies. It is interesting to note, however, that the lowest of the range of figures reported by Denhoff is a considerable increase over the California figure. What accounts for this disparity is unknown, but advances in medical technique have been made to the extent that more of these children are surviving to an age of diagnosis and classification.

The floppy child. Several authors have reported the presence of atonia or hypotonia in infancy (a lack or diminished level of muscle tone) as a part of the cerebral palsy complex. This child, with soft, flabby muscles, most often does not develop cerebral palsy (Jones, 1975b); however, it has been reported that the floppy child with a characteristic lack of muscle tone, may later develop signs of other types of involvement (Bartram, 1969), including a form of the spastic type of cerebral palsy (Bleck, 1975). Bleck's statement that "atonia is nonexistant in school children" (p. 44) should be considered within the realm of more traditional school settings and the requisite age groups within the schools. Educational opportunities are being offered to even lower chronological age levels in an effort to provide early identification and services that might work towards the reduction or alleviation of disability symptoms. Hence, in infant schools and treatment settings, teachers may well come into contact with the child who has poor muscle tone: the floppy child.

Topographical classification

In addition to the classification of cerebral palsy that describes the motor characteristics by identified type—spasticity, athetosis, and so on—, other formats need to be considered to bring a more definitive picture of the physical involvement of the individual. An additional classification involves topography, or the area of the body where the motor problem is located. Minear has suggested that a discussion of body topography include:

Monoplegia: Involvement of one limb.

Paraplegia: Involvement of the lower limbs. This classification is most often associated with the spastic type. (Another classification sometimes used is that of diplegia—involvement of the same parts on both sides of the body—bilateral involvement.)

Hemiplegia: Involvement of one side of the body. This classification is most often associated with the spastic type.

Triplegia: Involvement of three limbs, usually both legs and an arm. Although this classification is most often associated with the spastic type, it is not a designation that is often made.

Quadriplegia: Involvement of all four limbs. Both spastic and athetotic types are included in this classification.

Although the above body area classifications refer to involvement particularly of the limbs, it should be understood that this reference is made to those areas that are most frequently used for motor control in such activities as walking, or grasping and releasing, and in other fine and gross motor activities.

Classification by degree of involvement

In terms of the description of the functional behavior of children with cerebral palsy who may be present in the classroom, the last classification system to be considered is the severity of the motor involvement. Although the terms used to describe the degree of involvement are easily recognized and used, they are not always mutually understood by all those who use them. The three degrees of physical limitation or involvement used for this discussion are *mild*, *moderate*, and *severe*. The level of difference between these terms may be dependent on the point of view of the person making the designation. A person who is wheelchair bound but who has complete use of the upper extremities may be classified as mildly involved. On the other hand, another person with the same degree of physical limitation may be referred to as moderately or even severely involved, particularly if that individual had been especially physically active before becoming wheelchair bound, or if the person making the judgement considers a high degree of physical activity necessary for personal success or life fulfillment.

Because these are, in fact, no more than highly subjective conclusions regarding individual functioning and expectations, a more concrete criterion needs to be employed. Although not very recent, Deaver's descriptions (1955) are still useful because of the explicitness of the activity level included in each category:

Mild: No treatment is needed. The individual has no speech problem, is able to care for self, and can walk without the aid of appliances.

Moderate: Treatment is needed for speech problems and/or difficulties in ambulation and self-care. Braces and other equipment are needed.

Severe: Treatment is needed, but the degree of involvement is at a level wherein the prognosis for speech, self-care, and ambulation is very poor.

Three points of particular interest might be noted with regard to the use of these classification terms. First, there is the determination of the need for some type of treatment in light of the involvement of the individual. Second, the descriptions assigned to each of the terms deal primarily with a specific kind of activity: ambulation, speech, and so on. There is an avoidance of technical aspects of functioning, such as strength and range of motion. Although these descriptions may appear to be of a general nature, the important feature about them is the use of activity of the individual as opposed to a measurement or clinical designation. The third point of interest is the use of a prognosis in the last of the categories. The same activities are considered in each of the categories; however, only in the last of these categories ("severe") is the potential for treatment outcome considered. Although the "moderate" designation refers to treatment for the improvement of levels of activity, there is a lack of prognosis associated with the treatment.

ETIOLOGY

The etiology of cerebral palsy is discussed at this juncture because to be able to put some order to the characteristic aspects of the physical components of the symptom set generally known as cerebral palsy—motor type, topography of involvement, and degree of involvement—it is first necessary to understand the relationship of brain damage to motor dysfunction. For the classroom teacher, however, the concerns of etiology may be of little more than academic interest in comparison with the characteristics a specific child may or may not present in functional behavior. The knowledge that a child may stumble and fall frequently because of a specific type of cerebral palsy that is at an identified level of severity is of considerably more importance than what caused the brain damage in the first place. Because of this relative distance from the concerns of the teacher, who is more responsible for and more responsive to the functional behavior of the child, the etiology of cerebral palsy is only briefly discussed.

In many instances, however, etiology has been utilized in the definition of cerebral palsy. A review of the definitions in the first part of this chapter will reveal that there is as much lack of conformity of etiological considerations in the definitions as there is in the rest of each definition. Cerebral palsy is, according to the collected definitions, caused by defect, injury, or disease; aberrant structure, growth or development; involvement; lesion; or other factors and events. When etiology is reviewed as a separate aspect of cerebral palsy, a basic feature that emerges is the time period in which the damage occurred. The two general time frames that are considered are *congenital* (present at or before the time of birth) and *acquired*.

Within the congenital period are subdivisions that are time referenced: *prenatal*—occurring before birth; perinatal—occurring shortly before birth (twenty-eighth week of gestation) to the first to fourth week after birth (Dorland, 1974); and *natal*—the birth period itself. Because of the obvious overlap of time between the prenatal and perinatal periods, this discussion focuses on the more generalized period of the prenatal time, followed by the natal—birth—period.

Problems that may cause damage to the brain during prenatal period include genetically transmitted occurrences (rare); maternal infection, such as rubella (German measles) during the first 3 months of pregnancy; maternal anoxia (lack of oxygen); trauma to the fetus; RH blood incompatability (infrequent today); harmful exposure to x-rays; maternal use of drugs; and maternal malnutrition (Minear, 1956).

The natal period—the birth process—is important in the etiological consideration of cerebral palsy. It is during this period that the infant will undergo considerable stress and potential for injury. Factors that may be associated with damage to the brain at birth include maternal and/or infant anoxia, prolonged delivery as well as its counterpart—precipitate birth, forceps delivery, pelvic or placental abnormalities, and breech birth (buttocks presentation). Other birth problems including the premature infant, might be included at this point. Although prematurity refers to the infant of low birth weight or shortened gestation period there is a relationship between this complication and cerebral palsy (Malamud and others, 1964).

The acquired brain damage, occurring in the postnatal period, includes many of the same causative agents of the congenital period: anoxia, direct trauma to the brain, and infections. Toxic causes, such as lead or arsenic poisoning, are also contributory to brain damage in the postnatal period. Vascular difficulties, though not common in children, and lesions to the motor areas of the brain from brain tumors and cysts are also causes of brain damage resulting in cerebral palsy (Minear, 1956).

When one considers the total number of cerebral palsy causes and uses the differential of congenital versus acquired forms one will find that the overwhelming majority of reported cerebral palsy cases is congenital (approximately 85%). The sex ratios for these two etiological forms are quite similar: in both instances, the male child is more frequently afflicted with cerebral palsy than the female child. Congenital form: boys 57%; girls 43%. Acquired form: boys 52%; girls 48% (Scherzer, 1974).

ASSOCIATED OR SECONDARY DISABILITIES

Cerebral palsy infrequently occurs as a single diagnositic entity. In the discussion on results of brain damage it is noted (Fig. 2-1) that there are several consequences possible in addition to cerebral palsy (motor dysfunction), including disturbances of intellect (mental retardation), speech and/or language problems, sensory losses, and disturbances of consciousness (epilepsy) or behavior. Reports vary regarding the number, types, and degree of the disabilities that often accompany cerebral palsy. As in other reports of incidence of disabilities or characteristics, the usefulness of the figures cited is somewhat limited because of the population variations and the variation from what might actually be found in any given

Table 4. Secondary disabilities to cerebral palsy

	Percentage of total reported population*				
Source of data	Mental retardation	Speech/language defects	Visual handicaps	Auditory defects	Seizures (epilepsy)
California survey, 1965-1966 (Gore and Outland, 1966)	32 (IQ unspecified)	38	6	5	9
Ingram, Jameson, Errington, and Mitchell (1964)	62-76 (IQ 50-90)	27-58	NR†	NR	30-42
Bleck (1975)	75	48	NR	NR	NR
Jones (1975)	NR	NR	60-80	33	33

*All figures are approximates based on calculations, estimates, or reports from the reported sources.
†Data not reported—may be unavailable or not conducive to present table categories.

classroom. The figures in Table 4 are provided simply as generalized and summarized data from several sources to indicate the wide spread of characteristics often seen with cerebral palsy.

Although the percentages vary widely in Table 4, there is sufficient data to support the notion that cerebral palsy is far from a single disabling occurence, and the figures seem, in some instances, to represent a very large incidence of multiple disability. These figures should be considered only in the light in which they are presented: examples of incidence figures. The dangers of generalization are well-known, and such generalizations as would be possible from these data would do a specific individual or class of children as much injustice as would the generalization of any group data to any other individual or group.

Mental retardation

The figures for mental retardation show variation depending on the levels of measurement used in determining IQ scores for mental retardation classification. In addition to the use of any specific measurement guide for determining the presence or absence of mental retardation, other considerations should be kept in mind: the ability of the child with a physical limitation or speech and/or language problem to respond adequately to test materials; the lack of environmental exploration of the child because of restricted movement and hence the possibility of failure in the development of a variety of concepts; and the comparison of test results of children with the limitations of cerebral palsy to the test results of a population used in establishing norms and test administration techniques. That there is potential for IQ scores to be measured in children with cerebral palsy is obvious.

In an effort to further an understanding of the intellectual functioning of the individual with cerebral palsy, the concept of *adaptive behavior*, is utilized in the definition of mental retardation accepted by the American Association on Mental Deficiency (Heber, 1961). The definition includes a functional aspect of mental ability so that *adaptive behavior* (maturation, learning, and social adjustment) becomes a guide for individuality and self-actualization. Although impairment of adaptive behavior may be used as an index of mental retardation, this index must also be considered in light of the experiential limitations of the child with cerebral palsy. The range of mental or intellectual measurement in a group of children with cerebral palsy is presented in Chapter 1 in the description of the characteristics of a school for children with physical disabilities. In summary of the issue of mental retardation as a secondary disability of cerebral palsy, the following is offered:

1. Some children with cerebral palsy have identified scores on tests of intelligence above the normal range.
2. Some children with cerebral palsy have identified scores on tests of intelligence within the normal range.
3. Some children with cerebral palsy have identified scores on tests of intelligence below the normal range.

Speech and/or language problems

The range of speech and/or language problems associated with cerebral palsy is as vast as the other characteristics of this disability. Speech capabilities of those with cerebral palsy range from the normal production of speech without any deficiencies to speech production so limited as to be nonfunctional for communication. Language deprivation may likewise range from normal reception processing and expression to that which is nonfunctional.

It is not surprising that speech impairments are a part of the cerebral palsy syndrome. Although speech production is, in part, a motor act and hence susceptible to impairment due to damage to motor-control areas of the brain, conditions of speech are also regulated and controlled by respiration, the muscles concerned with pharyngeal and laryngeal functions, and the parts of the mouth. Malfunctioning of any of these mechanisms may cause a variety of speech production disorders in articulation, rhythm, or quality.

The characteristics of speech pattern disorders are associated with the several types of cerebral palsy (Lencione, 1976). Keeping in mind the varying degrees of involvement, one may note that speech impairment of the two major types of cerebral palsy, spasticity and athetosis, is characterized by:

Spastic speech: "Slow, labored rate, lack of vocal inflection, gutteral or breathy quality of voice, uncontrolled volume, and, most important, grave articulatory problems which reflect the inability to secure graded, synchronous movements of the tongue, lips, and jaw" (Berry and Eisenson, 1956, p. 357).

Athetoid speech: "The speech of the athetoid presents varying gradations of a pattern of irregular, shallow, and noisy breathing; whispered or hoarse phonation, and articulatory problems varying from the extremes of complete mutism or extreme dysarthria [impaired articulation] to a slight awkwardness in lingual movement" (Berry and Eisenson, 1956, p. 358).

Speech and/or language development may be delayed because of neuromotor problems, limitations in concept development, impairment of hearing, and the presence of mental retardation. These factors, along with a lack of motivation on the part of the child, whose feedback from attempts at vocalizations may be less than totally rewarding, combine to add yet another dimension to the child whose thoughts and feelings are unexpressible or unintelligible because of physical limitations: frustration. Where the lack of communication may be impaired because of physical limitations, the frustrations experienced with efforts toward expression and the perceived impatience or intolerance of others may have the effect of creating an abstinence of thought and action to a degree that severely limits self-potential regardless of the state of capacity.

Sensory losses

Hearing loss in children with cerebral palsy is a frequent enough occurrence to require attention by those responsible for the education and treatment of these children with multiple disabilities. Although there is no specific type of hearing loss unique to cerebral palsy (Nober, 1976), there are hearing losses that occur with a high level of incidence, particularly when the types and etiology of cerebral palsy are considered together. Vernon's study (1970) of a population of children who were both cerebral palsied and deaf found that the RH factor, meningitis, and prematurity—etiological factors of cerebral palsy—were responsible for the occurrence of deafness. "All cases resulting from complications of RH factors were athetoids. Those with a history of meningitis were all hemiplegics. Prematurity, rubella, and unknown etiologies resulted in mixed forms of palsy" (p. 748).

Several advances in medical care are reflected in the population changes of children with cerebral palsy who are deaf. Because of the capability for preventing RH incompatibility—the leading cause of cerebral palsy accompanied by deafness—a reduction in the number of children with this combination of disability can be expected (Morris, 1973; Vernon, 1970). Other advances in medical care, have, however, increased the potential for children with this combined disability. In the past, many children who suffered from meningitis or the effects of maternal rubella during pregnancy did not survive beyond infancy. Today, many of these children survive and reach school age.

School placement for children with cerebral palsy who are deaf may be complicated, not only because of the motor involvement and hearing impairment and its consequent language and speech deficiences, but also because of a reported incidence of visual problems (Vernon, 1970) and the high probability of mental retardation. Children with a mild-to-moderate degree of motor involvement are usually placed in school programs for the deaf and hard of hearing, whereas the child with a more severe degree of physical impairment who is also mentally retarded is assigned to a school for children with physical disabilities.

Regardless of the school placement, several problems directly associated with the characteristics of the two disabilities are evident: the motor involvement of the cerebral palsy component, depending on the degree of limitation, may interfere with the production of appropriate speech for which auditory feedback is limited; and the physical involvement may also hinder the use of both the fine and gross motor movements of the fingers and hands in the finger-spelling and signing forms of communication advocated by some special schools and classes for the deaf (Vernon, 1970). For the child who is placed in a school or class for children with physical disabilities, acoustic conditions in these classes may prove to be detrimental to speech discrimination. Factors such as increased noise levels as a result of the awkward, uncontrolled, involuntary movements of children; the use of wheelchairs and other walking aids; and the movement of furniture to ease standing and sitting at desks provide for excessive noise levels and overall poor environmental conditions for the learning and utilization of speech (Morris, 1973).

Visual impairments often seen with cerebral palsy may be divided into three major types: ocular muscle dysfunction, refractory errors, and perceptual problems. Of the problems related to muscle dysfunction, the two most common are strabismus and nystagmus. Strabismus is the condition often referred to as "cross eyes," wherein the two eyes are not in normal alignment. "Usually one eye fixates and one deviates, but both may be affected" (Cardwell, 1956, p. 333). Nystagmus, less common in children with cerebral palsy than strabismus, is characterized by a seemingly constant motion of the eyes, which may vary from a rapid, jerky motion of the eyeball to slower involuntary motion (Cardwell, 1956).

Refractive errors of vision, those associated with the acuity or clearness of vision, are common visual defects found in children with cerebral palsy. Twice as many children with the spastic type of cerebral palsy have visual acuity defects (both hyperopia—farsightedness—and myopia—nearsightedness) as compared to children with the athetotic type, who are more often farsighted (Capute, 1975).

In addition to the visual problems mentioned above, the visual-perceptual problem is one of considerable importance to the teacher. Just as the muscle and refractive errors become the treatment domain of the opthamologist, problems of impaired visual perception become the concern of the classroom teacher. Such defects as form discrimination, foreground-background problems, and visual-motor coordination provide significant problems to the learning of reading, writing, and other academic or learning skills.

Other problems concerning the development of the child with cerebral palsy who is visually impaired are related to the degree of involvement; for the child who has a visual loss to the degree that print becomes nonfunctional for learning, problems associated with the use of low-vision aids such as magnifiers, the management of large-print books, the use of auditory aids for learning, and the ability to learn and use braille become of paramount importance to the teacher. These problems of learning are further complicated by the restriction of mobility that is imposed on the child whose visual impairment may be at such a level that vision needed for travel is inadequate. The lack of vision for travel and the varying degrees of physical limitations combine to make environmental orientation and physical mobility a monumental task for the child who has cerebral palsy and is severely visually impaired or blind.

Seizures or epilepsy

Epilepsy often is thought of in terms of its manifestations: seizures. Many children with cerebral palsy have seizures, which, in addition to the behavior exhibited during the seizure activity, may interfere with the learning process. Although the cause of epilepsy is not clearly established, it may be of a genetic nature (idiopathic) or it may be related to brain damage (Denhoff and Robinault, 1960). There are several seizure types; of these, the two most common are the petit mal and grand mal seizures.

The petit mal seizure may go unnoticed by the casual observer. This seizure, which is not common in cerebral palsy (Denhoff, 1976), is characterized by an interruption of activity, such as speech, reading, or writing, and may be further recognized by a fixed stare. This lack of consciousness lasts a short time and is of little or no particular danger to the individual.

The grand mal seizure is more serious in that it is generally of a longer duration than the petit mal type, and the possibility of physical harm to the individual is greater. Depending on the severity of the seizure, there is a lack of balance, causing the individual to fall, and a general writhing of the body and its extremities. Saliva forms in the mouth and appears on the lips; it is sometimes mixed with a small amount of blood, caused by the individual's biting of the tongue. This type of seizure lasts a minute or two and is further characterized by a complete lack of consciousness. Some individuals who have grand mal seizures have a warning sign (aura) of the impending seizure. The aura may be a tingling sensation or a sound or smell.

The implications for the teacher of the child who may have seizures is related to what the teacher can do during the time of the seizure and to the medication that is used to reduce the occurrence of the seizures or to lessen their magnitude. As mentioned on p. 40, the teacher and children in a classroom may be unaware of the petit mal seizure. In some cases, these seizures occur so infrequently or with such rapidity that they go completely unnoticed. The child who experiences the grand mal seizure is best served by the teacher remaining calm and trying to make the child as comfortable as possible during the seizure activity. If the child has an aura and can let the teacher know of an impending seizure, the teacher may have time to help the child into a comfortable position where the child will not harm him/herself during the physical activity associated with this type of seizure. Moving furniture and protecting the child's head are actions the teacher can take to help reduce the possibility of the child being injured during the seizure. The teacher should not try to place anything between the teeth of the child before or during the seizure as protection against biting or swallowing the tongue. The possibility of injury to the child or to the teacher during such a maneuver may prove to be more harmful than the child's biting of the tongue. After the conclusion of the seizure, the teacher should provide a place for the child to rest, since the child is likely to be tired from the physical activity of the seizure.

The teacher also needs to be aware of the medication used in the treatment of the seizures. The overall result of medication for seizures is the reduction of seizure activity in the child. A secondary effect not under the control of the teacher but involving the teacher is that anticonvulsant drugs may depress the functioning level of the child. It has been cautioned that in the very young infant an excess of sedation may result in a "deprivation of experience" and hence reduce the learning potential of the child (Jones, 1974, p. 32). Although caution needs to be taken in generalizing from this statement to the effects of medication on older school children, experience has shown that this experience deprivation may be noticed in older children.

THE CHILD WITH CEREBRAL PALSY

Cerebral palsy has been presented as a collection of types, conditions, and characteristics. A child might be described as having severe athetosis quadriplegia with moderate speech involvement, some loss in hearing, a deficit in tactile sense, and occasional grand mal seizures; he/she might be functioning intellectually at an educable mentally retarded level. A closer look at this description of a child with multiple disabilities will reveal the use of a large amount of terminology with little or no description of the child beyond it. An exercise that would bring into focus the child rather than the terms used to label and categorize him/her would be to describe the child's functional behavior without using these terms. Although the terms of classification may indicate a generalization of function, they also serve to deemphasize the characteristics of the individual. Each of us should strive to recall the human factor in our interactions with children.

TREATMENT CONSIDERATIONS

The last spoke on the wheel of cerebral palsy depicted in Fig. 2-1 is that of treatment considerations and includes activities related to the various problems that may be associated with this disability. No child should ever be viewed alone. The child's relationship with his/her parents, teachers, therapists, and physicians must form an integrated whole in order for the child to derive the maximum benefits from intervention.

The teacher's role in treatment is most directly related to the educational domain, whereas other aspects of management may be in the hands of physicians, therapists, and so on. Although special education practices and the functions of other treatment specialists are discussed elsewhere, it may be of some merit to discuss the concerns and goals for management or treatment of the child with cerebral palsy. All of the persons concerned with the care and treatment of the child establish goals for their own treatment process or procedure. Therefore, it is not unlikely that there may appear goals for surgery, goals for therapy, educational goals, and goals related to the vocational potential of the child. An examination of the types of goals or aims for the child by these various individuals would draw attention to the overlap and, at the same time, the hope that the child will be able to perform at his/her maximum potential. Primary goals for the child, which may serve as a base for other, more individually determined directions, might include the ability:

> To eat in a socially acceptable way
> To dress including choosing attire, without assistance
> To become mobile without assistance and with the least possible prosthetic support
> To make decisions, i.e., to make rational selections between meaningful alternatives
> To contribute in some significant way to the society in which they live
> To interact with other individuals for their mutual benefit (Jones, 1974, p. 19)

Jones (1975a) has suggested that the experiences that are a part of the growing child's development are directly related to personality traits that will identify the individual character in later life. These traits include the ability to accept oneself, to accept criticism, and to establish realistic goals. The importance of these and other traits should not be taken lightly or for granted. These goals and traits are not particularly unusual or uniquely different from those of persons who might be considered able-bodied or normal. What brings special importance to these statements of life expectancies are the interventions that are required to raise the individual above the social and psychological restrictions imposed by self or by others.

When considering these statements regarding what might be reasonably expected for a handicapped individual's growth and development, one must keep in mind that these goals are most often identified and enumerated by others. Although they are made in the best interests of all concerned, there may be some dissonance between these goal statements and the statements of rights and expectations that have been developed by and for those with disabilities. What is expected behavior by some may be deemed an infringement of rights by others or even a restriction of expression of rights. Such discrepancy is an obvious outcome when one group establishes goals for the benefit of another group, regardless of the number of times these goals are reviewed and revised because of some assumed or real progress and improvement of personal attainment. The basic concern is for self-determination within the capability for making such a determination. Persons with cerebral palsy are, in aspects of human dignity and rights, not unlike all the others who would set them apart.

SUMMARY

Cerebral palsy is one of the several resulting conditions that may be attributed to brain damage. Damage to the specific motor areas of the brain result in a variety of clinical types of cerebral palsy with varying degrees of severity and different areas of body involvement. In addition, cerebral palsy may be accompanied by other disabilities, including mental retardation, speech impairments, disorders of perception and sensory functioning, and epilepsy.

One must take care not to generalize cerebral palsy by using a label such as "CP" or "the spastic child" or any other in which the person's individuality is lost or denied. The range of characteristics of the disability, the treatment processes available, and the special, unique qualities of each individual preclude any reliable generalization. Teachers must first and foremost be concerned with the child as he/she functions and performs in the classroom. A preconceived notion of what the child ought to be able to do and not be able to do makes one blind as to what the child actually can and cannot do.

REFERENCES

Bartram, H. B. Cerebral palsy. In W. E. Nelson (Ed.), *Textbook of pediatrics*. Philadelphia: W. B. Saunders Co., 1969.

Berry, M. F., and Eisenson, J. Speech disorders. New York: Appleton-Century-Crofts, 1956.

Bleck, E. E. Cerebral palsy. In E. E. Bleck and D. A. Nagel (Eds.), *Physically handicapped* children, a medical atlas for teachers. New York: Grune & Stratton, Inc., 1975.

Capute, A. J. Cerebral palsy and associated dysfunctions. In R. H. A. Haslam and P. J. Valletutti (Eds.), *Medical problems in the classroom.* Baltimore: University Park Press, 1975.

Cardwell, V. A. *Cerebral palsy, advances in understanding and care.* Baltimore: The Williams & Wilkins Co., 1956.

Deaver, G. G. Cerebral palsy: methods of evaluation and treatment. *The Institute of Physical Medicine and Rehabilitation,* 1955, 9.

Denhoff, E. Medical aspects. In W. M. Cruickshank (Ed.), *Cerebral palsy, a developmental disability.* Syracuse, N.Y.: Syracuse University Press, 1976.

Denhoff, E., and Robinault, I. P. *Cerebral palsy and related disorders, a developmental approach to dysfunction.* New York: McGraw-Hill Book Co., 1960.

Dorland's illustrated medical dictionary (25th ed.). Philadelphia: W. B. Saunders Co., 1974.

Gore, B. E., and Outland, R. W. *Incidence report on types of handicaps found among children enrolled in special day schools for the orthopedically handicapped including the cerebral palsied in California (1965-66 school year).* Sacramento: Department of Education, State of California, 1966.

Heber, R. Modification in the manual on terminology and classifications in mental retardation. *American Journal of Mental Deficiency,* 1961, 46, 499-501.

Ingram, T. T. S., Jameson, S., Errington, J., and Mitchell, R. G. *Living with cerebral palsy, a study of school leavers suffering from cerebral palsy in Eastern Scotland.* London: William Heinemann Medical Books, Ltd., 1964.

Jones, M. H. Diagnosis and general assessment in cerebral palsy. In M. Hoffer and P. H. Pearson (Eds.), *Syllabus of instructional courses,* American Academy for Cerebral Palsy, 28th Annual Meeting. Washington, D.C.: The American Academy for Cerebral Palsy, 1974.

Jones, M. H. Cerebral palsy. In R. M. Peterson and J. O. Cleveland (Eds.), *Medical problems in the classroom, an educator's guide.* Springfield, Ill.: Charles C Thomas, Publisher, 1975. (a)

Jones, M. H. Differential diagnosis and natural history of the cerebral palsied child. In R. L. Samilson (Ed.), *Orthopedic aspects of cerebral palsy.* London: William Heinemann Medical Books, Ltd., 1975. (b)

Keats, S. *Cerebral palsy.* Springfield, Ill.: Charles C Thomas, Publisher, 1965.

Lencione, R. M. The development of communication skills. In W. M. Cruickshank (Ed.), *Cerebral palsy, a developmental disability.* Syracuse, N.Y.: Syracuse University Press, 1976.

Malamud, N., Itabashi, H. H., and Castor, J. Etiologic and diagnostic study of cerebral palsy. *Journal of Pediatrics,* 1964, 65, 270-293.

Minear, W. L. A classification of cerebral palsy. *Pediatrics,* 1956, 18, 841-852.

Morris, T. Hearing impaired cerebral palsied children and their education. *Public Health,* 1973, 88, 27-33.

Nober, E. H. Auditory processing. In W. M. Cruickshank (Ed.), *Cerebral palsy, a developmental disability.* Syracuse, N.Y.: Syracuse University Press, 1976.

Perlstein, M. A., and Hood, P. W. Etiology of post-neo-natally acquired cerebral palsy. *Journal of the American Medical Association,* 1964, 188, 850-854.

Scherzer, A. L. Early diagnosis, management, and treatment of cerebral palsy. *Rehabilitation Literature,* 1974, 35, 194-199.

Vernon, M. Clinical phenomenon of cerebral palsy and deafness. *Exceptional Children,* 1970, 36, 743-745.

3 Musculoskeletal disabilities and other health impairments

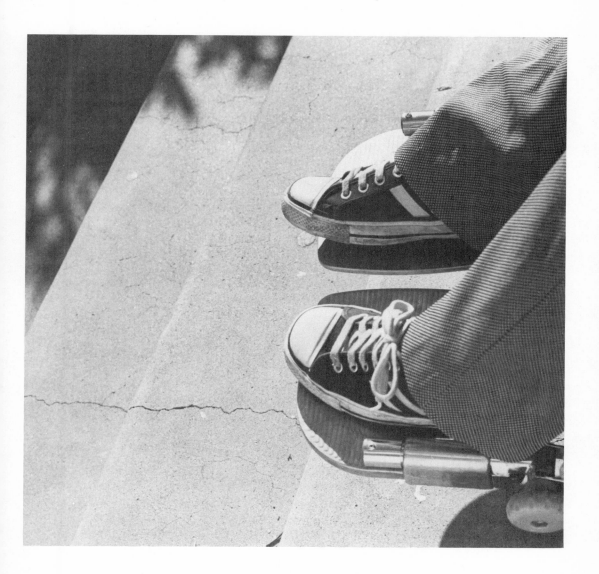

A discussion of the many and varied disabilities that may be found in a classroom of children with physical disabilities is dependent on several factors. In addition to the selection of disabilities to be discussed, consideration should be given to describing the disabilities in such a manner as to be accurate and yet not so clinical as to draw attention to the disability rather than to the person with the disability. There is also a need to concern oneself with the other characteristics of the individual's disability that may be as important to the understanding of and response to this person as are the physical characteristics: the implications of the disability on the individual for learning, the individual's adjustment, and the parental response. The choice of disabilities described here is arbitrary and not related to specific ratios in any given population of children with disabilities or according to any format reflecting one disability as being more important or more disabling than another.

Two major classifications of disabilities are presented here: *orthopedic disabilities* (disabilities relating to the structural—skeletal and muscular—capacity of the individual to maintain him/herself in a straight and normal condition) and *health impairments* (disabilities that, although not visually obvious, nonetheless restrict the physical well-being, health, and physiological functioning of the individual).

It should be made clear that the list of disabilities described here is far from exhaustive and may only, in the most biased of populations, be representative of disabilities seen in classes and schools for children with disabilities. That there are disabilities that the reader will not find described here is obvious. What is not quite so obvious is the importance attached to listing any disabilities at all. It is only with a great deal of reluctance that the topic of disability characteristics is even pursued, since this phenomenon is probably of least significance in the interaction with the *person*.

The amount or extent of knowledge about a disability that the teacher should have may be reduced to two levels: the requirements of the child for safe, comfortable, functional physical behavior that is not contradictory to medical treatment or growth and development; and the physical and behavioral concomitants that are necessary for learning and for functioning in school. The remainder of what there is to know about children with various disabilities is no different from the knowledge required by *any* teacher in fulfilling his/her duties and responsibilities in *any* classroom.

ORTHOPEDIC DISABILITIES
Amputations

Amputation refers to the absence at birth or to the removal at a later time of a limb or limbs, or parts thereof. The discussion of amputations is unique in that this particular orthopedic disability is one in which there are two etiological possibilties: the condition is present at birth (congenital) or the amputation occurs after birth. The dichotomy of the two conditions is particularly meaningful with regard to physical growth, development, and functioning and with regard to the psycho-social implications. Congenital anomalies, or malformation, of the extremities are not uncommon, occurring in 2% to 3% of newborns (Swanson and Glessner, 1964), and account for the overwhelming majority of amputations in children (aged 0 to 10). Alexander (1975) has reported an incidence ratio of 75% and 25%, respectively, for the congenital and later occurring types. The causes of amputations after birth range from traumatic injuries (automobile or railway accidents, for example), which account for 68% of these amputations, to the effects or results of disease states.

Congenital-type amputations occur because of failure of the limb to develop properly during the early stages of gestation (Bleck, 1975a). These may take the form of total absence of a limb or limb part or of multiple anomalies, including the absence of limb parts and/or malformation of limbs, as in the case of the congenital amputations that have been related to the use of thalidomide by mothers during pregnancy. The limb deformities of the congenital-type amputation are identified by the site and type of deficiency, such as amelia (absence of a limb or limbs) or phocomelia (a malformed hand or foot with abnormal attachment at the shoulder or pelvis); other anomalous limb formations may include the presence of a normal limb part with an abnormal formation at a knee or elbow joint or at another level of the extremity (d'Avignon, Hellgren, Juhlin, and Atterback, 1967).

Amputations because of trauma or disease complications are described by the level of amputation of the limb: above the knee or below the knee (sometimes referred to as AK or BK) and above the elbow or below the elbow (AE or BE) (Lambert, Hamilton, and Pellicore, 1969). Amputation levels may also include shoulder, wrist, and hip disarticulations as well as other levels and degrees of loss (Blakeslee, 1963; Bleck, 1975).

Limb replacement through artificial means—a prosthesis—is dependent on a variety of characteristics of the child with the amputation: the age of the child, the type and level of amputation, the psychological adjustment of the child to his/her disability, the support of the family, and the need for the device. Similarly, prosthetic design fitting and function are related to the type and level of amputation and to the function of the limb for which the prosthesis is substituted. The importance of this may be appreciated when one considers the presence or absence of a natural joint in the functioning of the limb. The range of motion of the normal elbow or knee is considerable; in comparison, the mechanical joint of the prosthesis has restriction of motion in several planes.

Upper-limb prothesis designs vary according to the level of amputation and may include a prosthetic elbow or shoulder, as well as a hand replacement or terminal device. The terminal device may be of two basic types: the hook type or the cosmetic hand (Garrett, 1975). The hook-type terminal device, which is operated by a cable attached to a shoulder harness, allows for grasp and release activities, and the individual can utilize the hook to gain and maintain support and balance in coming to a sitting and standing position. The cosmetic hand may or may not be functional; its main feature is in its approximation to normal appearance.

Lower-limb prostheses require considerations in design and function similar to those of upper-limb prostheses; they also vary according to the level and type of amputation. In addition to these obvious considerations, there is also the problem of functionalism in relation to locomotion. Whether the amputation is unilateral or bilateral, above the knee or below the knee, the problem of bearing weight on the stump for ambulation and the requirements of foot motion for balance and walking are of major concern.

One of the important considerations in the fitting of the prosthesis to the child is related to the age of the child. The prosthesis should be fitted to the child with the goal of assisting the child through the normal developmental stages in a manner as close to normal as possible (Alexander, 1975). A lower-limb prosthesis may be used when the child begins to attempt standing balance, and an upper-limb prosthesis may be used when the child attains sitting balance (Aitken and Frantz, 1964; Garrett, 1975). In addition to the functional aspects of a prosthesis, the wearing of one may aid in the development of body image, self-confidence, and competence; these may be nurtured in the child through the early fitting and training of the prosthesis and through professional and familial support.

Prostheses for children in whom amputations have occurred after birth may vary little from those used by children with congenital-type amputations. In both cases, the prosthesis is individually prescribed and designed to accommodate the nature of the amputation and stump characteristics. With the second type of amputation, the time at which a prosthesis may be fitted to the child following surgery is dependent on the stump condition and the healing process required.

Associated problems that may occur with amputations are as varied as the individuals with the amputations, the degrees and conditions under which the amputations have occurred, and the response of others to the person and his/her disability. The teacher of a child with an amputation may need to be particularly aware of such physical problems as skin breakdown from improper wearing or use of the prosthesis; mechanical problems of broken cables, harnesses, or other device-oriented problems; or an unwillingness on the part of the child to wear the prosthesis. Attention should also be given to adjustment problems of the child and the parents at various developmental stages; these may range from initial confrontation of the disability through and including personal self-image changes accompanying adolescence and young adulthood. The educational implications surrounding the use of materials in the classroom should also be considered. Activities that may require training and skill of the child in the use of his/her prosthesis include writing, page turning, and other fine-motor activities and playground and recreational activities such as the use of bats, balls, and other play equipment.

Arthrogryposis

Arthrogryposis multiplex congenita, often called simply arthrogryposis, is a congenital condition with an unknown cause. A simple definition of arthrogryposis has been proposed by Friedlander, Westin, and Wood (1968); according to them, arthrogryposis is a syndrome of persistent joint contractures present at birth. A description of this condition that may belie this rather noncomplex definition include the location of the involvement, the amount of fixation, and the degree of involvement. Several causes have been postulated for this condition, including mechanical abnormalities and abnormalities of the central nervous system (Friedlander and others, 1968). Bleck (1975b) has suggested that the condition may be the result of a lack of early movement of the joints during fetal development; however, Bleck also states that the condition is not hereditary. This latter fact becomes important in the counseling of the parents of the child with arthrogryposis.

Involvement includes various sites of the body, and different degrees of involvement are present according to the amount of rotation of the body parts and the location of the movement attempt (Michele and Eisenberg, 1967). Body part involvement includes inwardly rotated shoulders, elbows and knees either fixed in extension or flexion, wrists fixed in a flexed position and turned inwardly, slender fingers curled into the palm, hips in flexion and with outward rotation, and feet and ankles turned in and down (Bleck, 1975b; Friedlander and others, 1968).

Three major groups of symptoms of arthrogryposis have been described (Weeks, 1967). The least involved group is that involving a single localized body part, such as the wrist or elbow; the group with the next level involvement is of a more generalized nature and includes deformity of several upper-extremity parts—wrist, arms, shoulders, and so on; the third group has the most severe level of involvement and includes deformity of both the upper and lower extremities.

Medical treatment of the child with arthrogryposis involves frequent and radical surgery (because of the reoccurrence of the deformities) and the use of a variety of casts, splints, and braces. Another treatment technique has been suggested by Hillman and Elmore (1966). They have proposed that involvement of the mother in "dynamic, prolonged manipulations" (p. 1652) of the child's extremities in the first months of life will help to reduce joint stiffness. This technique, which includes training of the mother, is a 6- to 8-hour-a-day commitment to treatment. Of particular significance to this technique is the active role of the mother in the treatment of her child. The implications are that physical and emotional energy output by the mother must be great, and readjustment to roles and expectations may be required for all family members.

The teacher's concern for the child with arthrogryposis is of particular importance, since "no matter how severely involved, [they] can be helped and many overcome their severe handicaps sufficiently to become useful citizens" (Friedlander and others, 1968, p. 111). Physical activities in the classroom or on the playground will be dictated by the level of involvement and the restrictions imposed by joint contracture, walking ability (some may be wheelchair bound), and the ability to manipulate the learning materials of the classroom. If they are not capable of using pencils or other writing tools, children with arthrogryposis may successfully use a typewriter and may participate in a variety of school activities, including drivers training and work training, that will lead to independent living activities and skills if selected by the child as within his/her interest and goal directions.

Legg-Perthes disease

Legg-Perthes disease (Legg-Calvé-Perthes disease, coxa plana, coxa plana juvenilis) is a disability that has been described as a self-limiting disease (Garrett, 1975) and is one that is most unusual among the disabilities seen in children with orthopedic problems. Legg-Perthes disease, named after the physicians who first described it, is transient in nature when treated and diagnosed at an early age of the patient. The transiency of this disease is represented through the disease course, treatment, and cure. When treatment is successful, the child is removed from the roles of individuals with disabilities.

Legg-Perthes is a disease of the head of the femur (growth center of the femoral head) of unknown cause. A lack of blood supply to this growth center of the femur results in disintegration and flattening of the femoral head at the hip joint. Weight-bearing pressure on the hip area results in a destructive process characterized by slight pain along the thigh and knee. The presence of this slight pain and limp are the first symptoms of the disease process.

This disease is most frequently seen in boys of elementary school ages; an approximate sex distribution is 80% males and 20% females (Fisher, 1972; Katz, 1967). The age of onset of the disease has been variously reported as "at or just before puberty" (Garrett, 1975, p. 196), "during the age period from 4-8 years" (Silberstein, 1975, p. 178), and between 3 and 12 years of age (Fisher, 1972). Although age specificity in detection is important, it is complicated by the possibility of the disease being undetected and unreported for as long as 6 months during the early stages of the disease process (Fisher, 1972).

Treatment success is particularly related to the age of the child, and the "prognosis is most favorable in the younger age group [although it] does not seem to be related to the duration of symptoms at the time of diagnosis or to the duration of therapy," (Katz, 1967, p. 1050). Treatment is aimed at reducing the weight-bearing pressure of the femoral head in order to eliminate the destructive process and to allow for bone restoration. Techniques used in treatment have been as varied as the several characteristic features of the disease itself. The three major reported treatments include bed rest; abduction bracing, which allows for ambulation, often with the required aid of crutches; and surgery involving the hip joint and femoral head (Cocchiarella, Challenor, and Katz, 1972; Eaton, 1967; Katz, 1967; Petrie and Bitenc, 1967). The length of treatment, though dependent on the type of treatment and the age of the child at diagnosis, may be 2 years or more. However, the surgical procedures, if appropriate, may reduce the healing process by 6 to 12 months (Silberstein, 1975).

The major concern for the special educator should be focused on the child's avoidance of physical activities that would put weight-bearing stress on the affected hip and on the child's continuation of the academic program. Given the conditions of early diagnosis and successful treatment, children with Legg-Perthes disease have an excellent chance of being able to participate in the activities of the normal population. The educational program, therefore, should be one that will enhance this prognosis and should be regarded, as with all children, as a link toward the development of independent adult living.

Muscular dystrophy

Of the several types of muscular dystrophy, the Duchenne type is both the most common and the most insidious. This is a disease wherein there is progressive and continuous weakening of the voluntary muscles of the body; the muscle cells are replaced by fatty, fibrous tissue. This progressive and degenerative disease has different characteristic features at the various stages of involvement. Although the child is born without any signs or symptoms of the disease, the first indications of involvement may occur by the age of 3 years. Zellweger and Hanson (1967) have identified ten stages of functional involvement, ranging from the first stage, when the child is still ambulatory and can climb stairs without railings, to the last stage, when the child requires bed confinement.

The progressive nature of the disease follows two avenues: progression related to the severity of involvement and progression of muscle group involvement. The disease advances from involvement of the pelvic-hip area to the upper extremities. The face, neck, and hand muscles are the last muscle groups to be involved. Severity of involvement through increased levels of muscle weakness reduce the functional ability of the individual to perform voluntary muscle activity. Death due to upper respiratory tract infection and/or cardiac failure may occur by the late teen years or early twenties. Life-saving techniques, including the use of antibiotics, have in many cases increased the life span of those with muscular dystrophy.

The physical activity characteristics that accompany the muscle group involvement include a swayback appearance (lordosis) with abduction and flexion of the hips as well as flexion of the knees (Siegel, 1972). This provides for an overall broader base for upright support, but walking becomes a clumsy tiptoe-appearing manuever. Increased muscle weakness causes increased awkwardness in walking, and frequent falls are noticed. When the child falls, "he gets up from the floor by walking up his thighs with his hand due to weakness of the thigh muscles" (Bleck, 1975c, p. 176). An inability to walk at all is seen by the time the child is 10 to 13 years of age.

In addition to activity restrictions, other body changes become apparent: enlarged calf and shoulder muscles and muscle contractions. In addition, weight gains are often reported, although Fowler and Gardner (1967) reported that only 30% of their study population showed marked obesity. This figure may vary among study populations, but the fact of weight gain creates significant problems for the parents, who must take on an ever-increasing role in the personal care of the child as the disease progresses. The additional weight makes dressing, toileting, bathing, turning the child in bed, and lifting the child in and out of the wheelchair very strenuous tasks. Although the use of portable hydraulic lifts may ease the task, the energy, stress and strain on both parent and child is considerable.

Duchenne-type muscular dystrophy is a sex-linked recessive-gene disease transmitted by a female carrier to her sons. It is rare for a girl to be identified with this type of muscular dystrophy, and this may occur only as the result of highly unusual genetic combinations (Fowler, Gardner, Taylor, Scavarda, and Busheikin, 1969). This information regarding genetic transmission becomes of extreme importance to the parents, who may seek genetic counseling and family planning, since the probability of more than one affected male offspring from the same parents is high.

Several educational implications are associated with muscular dystrophy. The presence of mental retardation in approximately one third of the population is of particular importance to the special educator in terms of educational planning and programming (Prosser, Murphy, and Thompson, 1969; Zellweger and Hanson, 1967). There is some question as to whether the mental retardation (IQ 75) is secondary to muscular dystrophy or is another variable of the disease. The work of Marsh and Munsat (1974) has suggested that the mental retardation found in some children with muscular dystrophy is neither totally nonprogressive nor uniform between verbal and performance abilities. According to their findings, the mental retardation is differentiated between verbal and performance abilities and the verbal ability is more involved than the performance ability. There does seem to be a reduction in the reported performance scores as the child grows older (and the subsequent involvement from the disease decreases physical ability). Some caution must be taken when interpreting test results, however, since the presence of the disease may cause the interpreter to underestimate the measured ability. Also, the level of progression of the disease at the time of intelligence measurement may play a significant part in the determining of an IQ when the test used contains both verbal and performance sections. Assumptions should not be made regarding the intellectual functioning of any child with muscular dystrophy at any stage of the disease.

Educational planning and programming for the child with muscular dystrophy, whether the child is functioning in the normal academic and intellectual range or not, should be done with care and with an eye toward the physical capabilities of the child. Classroom and playground activities requiring gross motor activities, strength, and stamina are inappropriate for this child, and adaptations of lessons to accommodate the child's physical limitations will be necessary.

Muscular dystrophy has an emotional impact on all those concerned; including family members as well as the child him/herself. The remembrance of things past, a normal infancy and early childhood, are in juxtaposition with the progression of weakness and disability and with the requirements of care and restriction of functioning in later years. The physical and emotional strain on the parents and siblings and the resentment that may be expressed by the child as the progressive nature of the disease becomes understood require compassion and support by the teacher. However, a maudlin overcompensation by the teacher should be avoided, and response to the child should be at the same level as that extended to other children in the class.

Osteogenesis imperfecta

Osteogenesis imperfecta, often referred to as brittle bones, is a disease in which there is an inborn error of connective tissue (Siffert, 1966) with consequent deficiencies resulting in bone structure weakness. Bleck (1975d) has stated that this is a dominant-gene inherited disease with occasional spontaneous occurrences without a familial history of the disease and that it is not disproportionately represented in either sex or in any race. Osteogenesis imperfecta has several characteristic features, including multiple fractures (which occur with less stress than would be expected to produce a fracture on a normal bone), deformity, dwarfism, hearing failure, a blue tint to the white of the eyes (blue sclerae), and a triangular facial appearance (Bleck, 1975d; Milgram, Flick, and Engh, 1973).

Two major types of osteogenesis imperfecta have been noted: (1) osteogenesis imperfecta congenita, which has a poor survival rate because of multiple fractures occurring before birth or in early infancy, and (2) osteogenesis imperfecta tarda, which may occur during early childhood. The tarda type of osteogenesis imperfecta has been reported to occur with two levels of involvement, which are based on the presence of bowing of the lower extremities. Tarda type I is characterized by bowing of the lower extremities, multiple fractures, and structural deformity; there is a good possibility for ambulation, but this activity may be late in occurring. Tarda type II, like tarda type I, has a very good survival rate; unlike either the congenital form or tarda type I, however, it does not involve bowing of the lower extremities and there are fewer fractures with less deformity, although the number of fractures and the degree of deformity are not predictable. The distinction between the two tarda types may be recognizable to the extent that an individual with tarda type II osteogenesis imperfecta may have a normal appearance, walk, and belie the fact of the diagnosis (Falvo, Root, & Bullough, 1974).

With the exception of the need to deal with a possible hearing loss that may accompany the disease, the educational implications for the child with osteogenesis imperfecta revolve around the physical activities of the child. The child needs to be discouraged and excluded from participation in activities that might result in bone fractures and encouraged to develop skills that will enhance his/her participation in other activities and areas of social contact. The educational program should include academic areas that will offer the individual a chance to pursue adult goals within his/her intellectual and physical capabilities.

Spinal canal defects

Three types of congenital spinal canal defects are frequently, and mistakenly, referred to interchangeably: spina bifida (spina bifida occulta), myelomeningocele, and meningocele. All three terms refer to an open defect of the spinal canal. Myelomeningocele refers to an exposed sac containing neural elements; meningocele refers to an exposed sac without neural elements within the sac; and spina bifida occulta refers to a defect without an external sac from the spinal column (Curtis, 1972a). It is the consequences of these defects that probably give rise to the common reference: "The potential for neurological deficit exists in any of the conditions listed in this classification and the musculoskeletal and urological problems we encounter are chiefly of paralytic origin" (Curtis, 1972a, p. 10).

These defects, which occur during embryonic development, may be associated with several characteristic problems to varying degrees: hydrocephalus (an enlarged head due to blocked circulation of cerebrospinal fluid within the brain); spinal curvature; lower limb involvement, including deformities of the ankles and feet; paralysis of the bladder and bowel, resulting in loss of voluntary elimination control; heart disorders; mental retardation; and psychosocial problems (Emery and Lendon, 1972).

Medical treatment for the child with these defects is directly related to the several accompanying problems of the defect. Shunts to drain cerebrospinal fluid from the brain may be used in the treatment of hydrocephalus; orthopedic surgery and bracing may be considered for deformities of the spine and extremities; careful treatment of urinary tract infections and training in the use and care of external urine collection bags for both the child and the parents may be required; bowel management through medication and diet will also involve the child and the parents; treatment for cardiac disorders and special education considerations relating to the presence of mental retardation are also of concern to specialists.

The overriding concern expressed by those who have written on the subject of myelomeningocele, including its related defects and the children, families, and professionals involved, is the psychosocial impact of the disease. Questions relating to the treatment and preservation of life and to the quality of life must be confronted (Lorber, 1972); consideration must be given to the stress of the parents on learning in the hospital of the birth of a child with a defect and their consequent need for comfort, information, and support regarding the care of their child and the preservation of the family structure. These family crises may increase with time because of the requirements of treatment: hospital visits, medical procedures, transportation costs, care for other children, trips for physical therapy, urine checks, diet regulation for bowel management, financial problems, marital problems, siblings' reactions, and finally, of prime importance, the needs of the child (Freeston, 1971).

The child experiences anxieties and concerns similar to those expressed by the parents, including concerns in regard to the child's functioning life-style, the stress of hospital visits, separation anxieties, self-confidence, knowledge about the disability, relationships with others both within and outside the family, and questions concerning the future and the role that the child will play in independent adult living.

At its most gloomy, the picture is one where the condition is associated with severe social isolation, frequent misery and depression, especially in girls, with problems of finding satisfying work or indeed any work at all, with preoccupying worries about the future and with the prospect of unfulfilled wishes in relation to marriage and children. (Dorner, 1976, p. 443)

Although the problems may seem insurmountable, the requirements for intervention have centered not around any specific problem but around the treatment team of specialists (Curtis, 1972b; Kummel, Lasoff, and Stockman, 1972). Although not a new concept, this treatment approach is essential for this disability because of the multiplicity and impact of the problems. In addition to the physician specialists and medical treatment specialists (physical and occupational therapists), the availability and utilization of a psychologist and social worker are of inestimable value.

Follow-up studies of children with myelomeningocele vary in their findings from reports of those who have survived to adulthood and who function at several levels of independence, including marriage and the bearing and rearing of children (Curtis, Butler, and Emerson, 1972), to reports indicating "a very reserved prognosis on an overall basis, even with the best of care" (Shurtleff and Foltz, 1972, p. 291).

For the special education teacher, concern must be directed toward the learning capabilities of the child, the question of mental retardation, and/or the problems often associated with poor school attendance because of hospital visits and other treatment requirements. In addition to these learning or school-related problems, the teacher of the child with spina bifida will need to be conscious of the physical needs of the child as they relate to bladder and bowel control. If the child is wearing an external urine collection bag, or if the child attends school wearing diapers, the teacher needs to be alert to the requirements of personal hygiene for the child, not only for cleanliness and infection control, but because of the social implications for the child if he/she is shunned by classmates as a result of odor or altered personal appearance. Care and patience in response to the needs of this child both academically and socially may result in a potential for a life-style in which positive self-confidence and independence are as attainable as they are for any other child.

Other orthopedic disabilities

A variety of other orthopedic disabilities may be found in classes for children with physical disabilities. These disabilities range from the once-common poliomyelitis (a viral infection accompanied by possible muscle paralysis) and rheumatoid arthritis (an inflammation of the joints, often painful and debilitating) to conditions not related to either a disease process or genetic deficiency or defect but to accidents, injury, or mistreatment of the child. In the latter instances, these children have suffered from trauma, the result of which is often pain and disfigurement or limited physical ability.

Burns, painful in acquisition and often painful in treatment, may result in disfigurement, which is particularly stressful for the individual if the burns are on the face, and in limited physical activity because of loss of body parts or function. In addition to the requirements of medical treatment and therapy, concern is also given to the self-image of the child and to the social consequences for the child and the parents.

Accidental injury resulting in temporary or permanent disability has increased dramatically in the past several years. Injuries from automobile and motorcycle accidents and from falls produce a variety of fractures and internal injuries that cover a wide range of disabilities and degree of involvement. Perhaps the most serious of these are spinal cord and brain injuries, which may result in paraplegic or quadriplegic paralysis. Loss of motor control, including ambulation, may be complete or partial, depending on the level and type of spinal cord involvement and the amount of brain damage. Further complications may include respiratory difficulties, loss of bowel and bladder control, and loss of sensation. Physical therapy and reeducation may be impaired by a lack of conceptual and/or perceptual ability as a direct result of injury or as a psychological consequence of acknowledging and dealing with the disability. These same conceptual and/or perceptual limitations may also interfere with educational management and goals.

Of growing concern to educators, medical personnel, and social workers is the number of children who are being treated for physical and emotional injuries as a result of child abuse and neglect. Physical injuries, including burns, fractures, and abrasions and contusions, are among those that, because of their severity, are causing children to be placed in hospital classes and in special education classes. Because the physical abuses of the child are a manifestation of the environmental complex in which the child and the parents are functioning, treatment includes working with the family, the child, and the forces that may be identified and controlled or changed.

HEALTH IMPAIRMENTS
Asthma

Asthma is a chronic health problem that has been reported as one of the major causes of school absences for children, particularly in the early years (Harvey, 1975; Mitchell and Dawson, 1973). Unlike other disabilities, the symptomatic characteristics of this disorder are not always present. A child having an asthma attack will develop a labored breathing pattern accompanied by wheezing that is often easily heard by others. The wheezing is the result of air escaping through the narrowed bronchial passages, which have been reduced in size because of the conditions precipitating the attack. In addition to the wheezing and labored breathing, respiration may be more frequent, and the child may develop a coughing episode during the attack. The occurrence of these attacks may be so infrequent as to allow for normal school attendance, or they may occur with such frequency that the child may be placed in a special school for children with physical disabilities or be taught at home by a visiting teacher.

Asthma is an allergic condition with other components that may precipitate an attack. The allergic reaction to environmental substances, which is found to run in families, may be accompanied by an emotional response. The labored breathing and other characteristic respiratory symptoms may become frightening to the child as well as to the parent, and the child may exhibit a great deal of emotional distress—crying, gasping, and so on—that in turn elicits a response from the parent, who may be anxious about the breathing patterns as well as the emotional distress of the child. A cycle is developed in which emotions not only play a part in the attack itself, but also may precipitate or complicate the attack.

For the teacher in the classroom, concern for the child who may be subject to asthmatic attacks should be centered around dealing with the child's frequent absences from school, reducing classroom conditions that may prove stressful to the child, and carefully supervising the amount and type of physical activity the child may engage in during the school hours. On the other hand, a child with asthma may rarely, if ever, have an attack at school. In this situation, the teacher should provide academic and social learning activities that will best develop in the child a growing sense of independence and success.

Cardiac disorders.

The walk from the front entrance of the school to the classroom and his/her desk may be an exhausting and trying part of the school day for the child with a cardiac disorder. Shortness of breath, fatigue, and sometimes a cyanotic appearance (blue appearance of the skin, particularly noticeable around the lips and fingers) are characteristics of the child with either congenital heart disease or an acquired heart disorder such as that associated with rheumatic fever.

Congenital heart disease, often associated with maternal rubella occurring during the first 3 months of pregnancy, is a complex and individual-specific type of disorder. Defects in the heart may be of several kinds, including holes in the walls of the heart chambers and various problems related to the flow of blood, involving the valves, arteries, and veins that connect the heart with the lungs and are responsible for carrying blood throughout the body.

The occurrence of a heart defect as a result of rheumatic fever is not seen as frequently today as in the past, because of the advances made in diagnosis and early treatment of rheumatic fever. Thus, not all attacks of rheumatic fever result in heart involvement; however, it is still the one characteristic of rheumatic fever that will persist after the attack has subsided.

Medical treatment for children with heart defects has made tremendous advances, and the field of infant cardiac surgery has resulted in the partial or complete correction of defects in 80% of children with congenital heart disease (Clarke, 1975). Because of these gains in treatment, the number of children with heart disorders in the special schools and classes is not as great as it once was. In addition, many children who have had successful surgical repair are now enrolled in regular educational facilities and are taking part in normal activities within the range of their physical stamina and well-being.

The teacher's concern for the child with a cardiac disorder in the classroom should be centered around two areas: the restriction of the child from physical exertion and activity that would precipitate distress and fatigue and the emotional impact of the disorder on the child and the family. In the case of the first area, the child's physician will be quite specific regarding the physical activity level appropriate for the child in the school setting. It is the responsibility of the teacher and others in the school to respect these requirements of the physician and not to let the protestations of the child succeed in subversion of these restrictions. In the case of the second area of concern, the teacher needs to be aware of the fears that may have been expressed by the parents for the child's well-being and of the fears that the child him/herself may express. Whether the child's fears are a result of personal experience or are a reflection of the parents' concerns and anxieties, they may result in a behavior pattern characterized by a withdrawing, self-protecting, and shy demeanor. The teacher may also see, on the other hand, an overreaction of the child to the protective, fearful, or anxious expressions of the parents; this over-reaction may be defiance of the restrictions implied or imposed on the child.

Hemophilia

Sometimes referred to as the bleeder's disease, hemophilia is a disease that may result in disabled physical functioning or be life threatening in severe cases as a result of severe trauma. This recessive-gene condition (mothers are carriers; half of their sons may be affected) is a blood disease in which coagulation is impaired. Because the clotting factor "variously known as anti-haemophilic factor (AHF), anti-haemophilic globulin (AHG), or factor VIII" (Rizza and Mathews, 1972, p. 452) is deficient, excessive bleeding may occur from the slightest cut or may even appear to occur spontaneously.

Despite the potentially severe complications resulting from this disease, several authors have suggested that the child with hemophilia may be expected to grow into adulthood and participate in a wide range of normal activities, including marriage and child rearing (Clarke, 1975; Leavitt, 1975; Myers, 1975). As with all disabilities, the amount of loss of physical function will be determined by the severity of the disease, the physical disability that may arise from the disease process, and the personal or social management of the individual involved.

The child with hemophilia may attend a regular school, depending on the degree of disability and treatment accessibility, or the child may attend a special school for children with physical disabilities. In either case, the teacher must be ever vigilant regarding the physical activity level of the child. Contact sports and activities with a potential for physical contact are to be avoided. The suggestion by Rizza and Mathews that children with hemophilia are not likely to bleed to death at school is of little comfort to either the child or the teacher if the child becomes injured at school. Boys who are afflicted with this disease may rebel at the physical restrictions imposed on them, and their reactions may range from self-protection and fear to a "chance it anyway" attitude toward participation in activities. If the "chance" does not result in injury, the risk may be repeated; injury from the activity may be responded to with anger and/or guilt.

The teacher needs to be aware of the medically allowed activity levels and the types of activities in which the child may participate. For the well-being of the child, the teacher will need to develop the technique of encouraging the child to be as active as possible and yet retain an awareness of an appropriate level of physical restriction.

Other health impairments

Several other health impairments may be represented in a classroom for children with physical disabilities. The frequency of their occurrence is highly variable, and the characteristics and degree of severity are also open to much variability. Diabetes, a disease in which there is an insufficient amount of insulin in the body, results in an overabundance of sugar in the system and a disturbed metabolism. The problems of diabetes for the child may be aggravated if he does not have a well-established dietary and insulin regimen, or if the treatment procedures are not well maintained. Cystic fibrosis, another disease that may be represented in the classroom, is a hereditary disease involving the lungs, pancreas, and other body organs. It is a progressive disease that is fatal in childhood, although some children are now surviving into adolescence and early adulthood (Myers, 1975). Lung damage from the defective functioning of the pancreas results in frequent coughing and the reoccurrence of respiratory involvement.

THE CHILD WITH MULTIPLE DISABILITIES: A VERY SPECIAL CHILD

This reference to the very special child with multiple disabilities is not made without careful consideration to the characteristics of the child and the impact of his/her special needs on the family and the teacher. This child, sometimes referred to as the multihandicapped child, the severely handicapped child, or the child with developmental disabilities, or by other terms implying a significant number and degree of problems, has a very special set of circumstances involving the etiology of the disabilities and his/her physical characteristics, behavioral patterns, growth and development, and potential for functioning.

A set of disability labels that might be used for a specific child might include, for example, cerebral palsy, congenital heart disease, mental retardation, visual and auditory and/or perceptual losses, speech and/or language deficiencies, sensation deficiencies, and social-emotional disturbances. This list is offered as an example only; these and other problems, with all their variations of degree or intensity of involvement, may or may not occur in any one child. When the immediacy of life support and maintenance are encountered and resolved (for however long a period is required), several questions must be dealt with: How can the child best learn, and grow and develop within his/her capabilities? How can the parents and the family best be encouraged to adjust and find room in their lives for the demands that will be made because of the needs of the child, and to deal with their own very special needs?

The complexity of learning will be a shared task involving the teacher, the parent, and the child. No assumptions can be made regarding the acquisition of skills, concepts, and responses in the child. To foster the learning process, the environment must be one that is developed or contrived to bring about the most success possible in a well-ordered manner. The teaching team, which should be composed of both the special education teacher and the parent, will need to plan and execute activities that will be sequentially developed and that will carry over from the school to the home and back again. The child will need to experience a structure to learning in which the concreteness of experience is followed by an abstract association.

Time, patience, structure, and love are the keys that will need to be retained and practiced if success is to be obtained in the child who has such a multiplicity of problems.

THE NEGATIVE VERSUS THE POSITIVE

It has been said, and not too infrequently, that we are a profession that seems to deal with negatives. Defects, diseases, abnormalities, and deficiencies are all on the negative side of the ledger. Is there *anything* positive that can be said about disability? About disability itself, there probably is little that can be said that would make one feel warm and good and have all the positive feelings one might like to have. But there *is* a balance side to the ledger and that is quite simply, *the children*.

SUMMARY

There are dozens of physically limiting conditions that might be represented in classes of children with physical disabilities. Orthopedic disabilities, including amputations, arthrogryposis, Legg-Perthes disease, and others, have been discussed. Health impairments limiting the ability of the individual to function in the environment, including asthma, cardiac disorders, hemophilia, and others, have also been identified and discussed. There has been no attempt to list all of the diseases and physical disabilities that may be found in any given population. Several good references are available to provide a more comprehensive review of the conditions that impair the functioning of children. Some of these, such as leukemia and other forms of cancer, may restrict the life span of the child; others, such as congenital anomalies of the musculoskeletal system, may hinder the active participation of the child in his/her growth and development.

This very limited discussion of disabilities should provide a point of departure for a more in-depth study of the many causes and characteristics of disability that may be found. The relevance here is not the number of disabilities presented, but the special qualities of those who are involved: the children.

REFERENCES

Aitken, G. T., and Frantz, C. H. The juvenile amputee: a fourteen-year follow-up. *Journal of Bone and Joint Surgery,* 1964, *46-A,* 1376.

Alexander, J. The child amputee: summary of a forum. *Archives of Physical Medicine and Rehabilitation,* 1975, *56,* 169-172.

Blakeslee, B. (Ed.), *The limb-deficient child.* Berkeley: University of California Press, 1963.

Bleck, E. E. Amputations in children. In E. E. Bleck and D. A. Nagel (Eds.), *Physically handicapped children: a medical atlas for teachers.* New York: Grune & Stratton, Inc., 1975. (a)

Bleck, E. E. Arthrogryposis. In E. E. Bleck and D. A. Nagel (Eds.), *Physically handicapped children: a medical atlas for teachers.* New York: Grune & Stratton, Inc., 1975. (b)

Bleck, E. E. Muscular dystrophy—Duchenne type. In E. E. Bleck and D. A. Nagel (Eds.), *Physically handicapped children: a medical atlas for teachers.* New York: Grune & Stratton, Inc., 1975. (c)

Bleck, E. E. Osteogenesis imperfecta. In E. E. Bleck and D. A. Nagel (Eds.), *Physically handicapped children: a medical atlas for teachers.* New York: Grune & Stratton, Inc., 1975. (d)

Clarke, R. R. Cardiac diseases. In R. M. Peterson and J. O. Cleveland (Eds.), *Medical problems in the classroom: an educator's guide.* Springfield, Ill.: Charles C Thomas, Publisher, 1975.

Cocchiarella, A., Challenor, Y., and Katz, J. F. Orthosis for use in Legg-Perthes disease. *Archives of Physical Medicine and Rehabilitation,* 1972, *53,* 286-288.

Cowie, V. Parental counselling and spina bifida. *Developmental Medicine and Child Neurology,* 1967, *9,* 110-112.

Cummings, V., and Molnar, G. Traumatic amputation in children resulting from "train–electric burn" injuries: a social-environmental syndrome? *Archives of Physical Medicine and Rehabilitation,* 1974, *55,* 71-73.

Curtis, B. H. Classification of myelomeningocele and congenital spinal defects. In American Academy of Orthopaedic Surgeons, *Symposium on Myelomeningocele.* St. Louis: The C. V. Mosby Co., 1972. (a)

Curtis, B. H. The team approach. In American Academy of Orthopaedic Surgeons, *Symposium on Myelomeningocele.* St. Louis: The C. V. Mosby Co., 1972. (b)

Curtis, B. H., Butler, J. E., and Emerson, C. C. Follow-up study of 100 patients over age 12 with myelomeningocele. In American Academy of Orthopaedic Surgeons, *Symposium on Myelomeningocele.* St. Louis: The C. V. Mosby Co., 1972.

d'Avignon, M., Hellgren, K., Juhlin, I. M., and Atterback, B. Diagnostic and habilitation problems of thalidomide-traumatized children with multiple handicaps. *Developmental Medicine and Child Neurology,* 1967, *9,* 707-712.

Dorner, S. Adolescents with spina bifida—how they see their situation. *Archives of Diseases in Childhood,* 1976, *51,* 439-444.

Eaton, G. O. Long-term results of treatment in coxa plana. *The Journal of Bone and Joint Surgery,* 1967, *48-A,* 1031-1042.

Emery, J. L., and Lendon, R. G. Neurospinal dysrhaphism syndrome. In American Academy of Orthopaedic Surgeons, *Symposium on Myelomeningocele.* St. Louis: The C. V. Mosby Co., 1972.

Falvo, K. A., Root, L., and Bullough, P. G. Osteogenesis imperfecta: clinical evaluation and management. *The Journal of Bone and Joint Surgery,* 1974, *56-A,* 783-793.

Fisher, R. L. An epidemiological study of Legg-Perthes disease. *The Journal of Bone and Joint Surgery,* 1972, *54-A,* 769-778.

Fowler, W. M., Jr., and Gardner, G. W. Quantitative strength measurements in muscular dystrophy. *Archives of Physical Medicine and Rehabilitation,* 1967, *48,* 629-644.

Fowler, W. M., Jr., Gardner, G. W., Taylor, R. G., Scavarda, A., and Busheikin, J. B. Quantitative measurements in female siblings and mothers of boys with Duchenne dystrophy. *Archives of Physical Medicine and Rehabilitation,* 1969, *50,* 301-310.

Freeston, B. M. An inquiry into the effect of a spina bifida child upon family life. *Developmental Medicine and Child Neurology,* 1971, *13,* 456-461.

Friedlander, H. L., Westin, G. W., and Wood, W. L. Arthrogryposis multiplex congenita, a review of forty-five cases. *The Journal of Bone and Joint Surgery,* 1968, *50-A,* 89-112.

Garrett, A. L. Orthopedic diseases. In R. M. Peterson and J. O. Cleveland (Eds.), *Medical problems in the classroom: an educator's guide.* Springfield, Ill.: Charles C Thomas, Publisher, 1975.

Harvey, B. Asthma. In E. E. Bleck and D. A. Nagel (Eds.), *Physically handicapped children: a medical atlas for teachers.* New York: Grune & Stratton, Inc., 1975.

Hillman, J. W., and Elmore, S. Arthrogryposis multiplex congenita. *The Journal of Bone and Joint Surgery,* 1966, *48-A,* 1652.

Hoffer, M., Ferwell, E., Perry, R., Perry, J., and Bonnett, C. Functional ambulation in patients with myelomeningocele. *The Journal of Bone and Joint Surgery,* 1973, 55-A, 137-148.

Katz, J. F. Conservative treatment of Legg-Calve-Perthes disease. *The Journal of Bone and Joint Surgery,* 1967, 49-A, 1043-1051.

Kummel, B., Lasoff, M. E., and Stockman, J. C. Management of spina bifida in a community hospital. *The Journal of Bone and Joint Surgery,* 1972, 54-A, 1568.

Lambert, C. N., Hamilton, R. C., and Pellicore, R. J. The juvenile amputee program: its social and economic value. A follow-up study after the age of twenty-one. *The Journal of Bone and Joint Surgery,* 1969, *51-A,* 1135-1138.

Leavitt, T. J. Hemophilia. In E. E. Bleck and D. A. Nagel (Eds.), *Physically handicapped children: a medical atlas for teachers.* New York: Grune & Stratton, Inc., 1975.

Lorber, I. Spina bifida cystica. *Archives of Diseases in Childhood,* 1972, *42,* 854-873.

Marsh, G. G., and Munsat, T. R. Evidence of early impairment of verbal intelligence in Duchenne muscular dystrophy. *Archives of Diseases in Childhood,* 1974, *49,* 118-122.

Michele, A. A., and Eisenberg, J. Arthrogryposis: its mechanism. *The Journal of Bone and Joint Surgery,* 1967, 49-A, 1244-1245.

Milgram, J. W., Flick, M. R., and Engh, C. A. Osteogenesis imperfecta, a histopathological case report. *The Journal of Bone and Joint Surgery,* 1973, 55-A, 506-515.

Mitchell, R. G., and Dawson, B. Educational and social characteristics of children with asthma. *Archives of Diseases in Childhood,* 1973, *48,* 467-471.

Myers, B. A. The child with a chronic illness. In R. H. A. Haslam and P. J. Valletutti (Eds.), *Medical problems in the classroom: the teacher's role in diagnosis and management.* Baltimore: University Park Press, 1975.

Petrie, J. G., and Bitenc, I. The abduction weight-bearing treatment in Legg-Calve-Perthes disease. *The Journal of Bone and Joint Surgery,* 1967, *49-A,* 1483.

Prosser, E. J., Murphy, E. G., and Thompson, M. W. Intelligence and the gene for Duchenne muscular dystrophy. *Archives of Diseases in Childhood,* 1969, *44,* 221-230.'

Raycroft, J. F., and Curtis, B. H. Spinal curvature in myelomeningocele: a natural history and etiology. *The Journal of Bone and Joint Surgery,* 1972, 54-A, 1335.

Rizza, C. R., and Mathews, J. M. Management of the haemophilic child. *Archives of Diseases in Childhood,* 1972, *47,* 451-462.

Shurtleff, D. B., and Foltz, E. L. Ten-year follow-up of 267 patients with myelomeningocele. In American Academy of Orthopaedic Surgeons, *Symposium on Myelomeningocele.* St. Louis: The C. V. Mosby Co., 1972.

Siegel, I. M. Pathomechanics of stance in Duchenne muscular dystrophy. *Archives of Physical Medicine and Rehabilitation,* 1972, 53, 403-406.

Siffert, R. S. The growth plate and its affections. *The Journal of Bone and Joint Surgery,* 1966, 48-A, 546-563.

Silberstein, C. E. Orthopedic problems in the classroom. In R. H. A. Haslam and P. J. Valletutti (Eds.), *Medical problems in the classroom: the teacher's role in diagnosis and management.* Baltimore: University Park Press, 1975.

Stark, G. D., Drummond, M. B., Paneprasert, S., and Roberts, F. H. Primary ventriculo-peritoneal shunts in treatment of hydrocephalus associated with myelomeningocele. *Archives of Diseases in Childhood,* 1974, *49,* 112-117.

Swanson, A. B., and Glessner, J. R., Jr. The treatment of congenital anomalies on the extremities by surgery and prosthetic replacement. *The Journal of Bone and Joint Surgery,* 1964, 46-A, 458.

Weeks, P. M. Surgical correction of arthrygpotic deformities of the upper extremity. *The Journal of Bone and Joint Surgery,* 1967, 49-A, 579-580.

Zellweger, H., and Hanson, J. W. Psychometric studies in muscular dystrophy type IIIa (Duchenne). *Developmental Medicine and Child Neurology,* 1967, *9,* 576-581.

4 Disability-related services

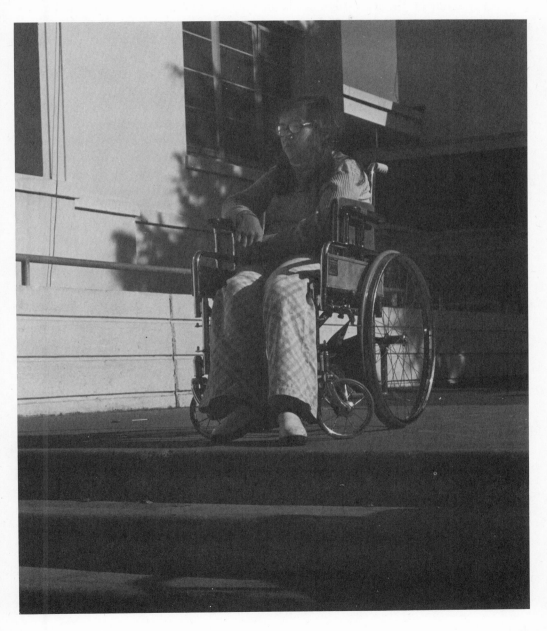

The services related to the treatment and education of the child with a physical disability are most often thought of in terms of the persons who offer or perform these services. These persons, working in conjunction with one another, usually have their own professional interests at the center of their approach to treatment. This may lead to a fragmentation of services or, at least, to a lack of coordination and a conflict of interests. Although certainly not a new concept in its approach to management, the *team approach* is the only one that fully contributes to the well-being and best interests of the child.

An analogy between the team interacting with the child and the family and the sports team may be appropriate when one considers the function of a team. In sports, the team consists of a group of players who have different functions or tasks to carry out in the prevention of an event (the opposing team making a score) and in the striving for other events to take place (scoring against the other team). The overall goal is to win the contest or event. When the team members act in such a way as to avoid reliance on a single feature or play or on the performance of a single player, then the effort that is expended is directed toward a unified goal: winning. When concentration is on a particular type of activity or play or on the skill of a particular individual, then the goal of the team may be lost; or at the very least, the team may lose sight of the goal.

Several similarities may be found between this sports team and the team interacting with the child and the family. The treatment team consists of several members who have different functions or tasks to carry out in the prevention of certain events (muscle contractures, the deterioration of physical and/or intellectual functioning) and in the striving for other events to take place (mobility within physical abilities, learning to accomplish academic tasks). The overall goal of the team involved in treatment has the same central feature as that of the sports team: maximum independence (in this case, the independence of the child). Whereas the sports team's goal is winning, the treatment team's goal is for the winner, the child. With individual treatments, or when individual team members participate at levels not consistent with the overall identified goal, the child may be lost or his/her achievement may lack unification of purpose and function. This should not be taken as a suggestion that there are not separate goals for each of the participants on the treatment team. It should, however, be recognized that the individual goals, as represented by the characteristics or modalities of treatment, should combine to reflect a total convergence of success for the child; they should not represent a collection of separate, but equal, goals. Although establishing the equality of the goals and their respective treatments is laudable, keeping them separate lacks a wholeness that is essential for reaching the overall team goal. Even though a single player or team member may function at the highest level, his participation must be in conjunction with the other team members for the result to be winning, rather than the recognition of individual player effort.

A true treatment team is a group of professionals working together—seeing, treating, following, making mistakes together, and learning to contribute and exchange views. This ultimately leads to a confluence of ideas. There should be no suppression of thinking, but rather a broadening of understanding that makes for better care. (Curtis, 1972, p. 301)

Curtis's perspective of the role and function of the treatment team is useful in focusing on the relationship of the team and its members to the care and services directed toward the child and the family. Team members and treatment services include a wide range of practices and professions, including physicians and their several specialities (pediatrics, orthopedic surgery, and cardiology, for example, and the subspecialities within each), physical and occupational therapists, speech therapists, social workers, psychologists, teachers, and a host of other specialists who may be essential for optimal care and development.

ROLE OF THE PHYSICIAN

To identify a team member simply as a physician is as inaccurate as referring to a member of a baseball team as a "player." Medical specialists with whom the school personnel are most likely to come into contact are the pediatrician and the orthopedist. The pediatrician, a physician whose professional concern is with the care and treatment of children, may be the primary physician in the school environment and the person responsible for recommending the child for placement in the school. This placement need not necessarily be in a special school. However, for special class or special school placement, the physician is required to make the judgment regarding placement based on the inability of the child to function with ease or safety in a normal school setting. In the past, a motivating factor in the physician's recommendation for placement of a child in a special facility was the presence of treatment facilities in the special school. These therapy services may be necessary for the physical habilitation or rehabilitation of the child and may not have been readily available at other sites. The practice today, whenever possible, is not to make a recommendation for placement in a special education facility solely for the purpose of having the child receive therapy if the child is capable of attending a regular school. The presence of outpatient treatment centers or of visiting or traveling therapists makes placement in a special school unnecessary.

The school pediatrician will most often see the child after the family pediatrician has made a recommendation for placement of the child in a special school or has referred the child for special medical treatment or therapy. On referral from the family physician, the school pediatrician will serve as a member of the team of specialists who will act as part of an admission-discharge committee for the child. This committee, composed of the pediatrician, occupational therapist, physical therapist, speech therapist, teacher, social worker, psychologist, school principal, and parents, will meet to evaluate the physical and educational characteristics of the child.

In the physical evaluation, the physician takes into account the total health development of the child, including a medical or health history and an examination to determine strong and weak areas of functioning, the extent of the disability, and the effects of the disability on functioning (Deaver, 1954). At this point, the pediatrician may have several recommendations for physical care, including referrals for further evaluation and treatment by the occupational and physical therapists or by the second of the physician specialists, the orthopedist.

The orthopedist, or orthopedic surgeon, who specializes in the functioning of the skeletal system, may advise surgical procedures or the use of braces or other appliances for the prevention of deformities or for the enhancement of motor activities.

> Surgery is generally indicated for those contractures that can be effectively released, those deformities which other measures have failed to bring to correction, and those for whom surgery is a preliminary step in preparation for subsequent treatment by the other modalities. In broad scope, the objectives of such surgery are the restoration of muscle balance, the realignment with bearing joints, and the establishment of a correct posture with normal relationship to the line of gravity. (Keats, 1970, p. 3)

The role of the physician in relation to the other members of the treatment team, including those members forming the educational component of the team, may become that of team coordinator; or the physician and the school administrator may become co-coordinators. The physician does not prescribe educational approaches, techniques, or directions, but does prescribe for the physical aspects of growth and development: occupational and physical therapy, orthopedic considerations, medication, and recommendations for the cessation of the various treatments when the child has reached a level of maximum function (Gottlieb, 1975).

Of primary importance in relation to the role of the physician in the care of the child and the family is the fact that the physician is a member of a team with a sphere of expertise and knowledge that is related to a specific set of characteristics of the child. In this regard, the physician is not unlike the other members of the team; it is through a collaboration of effort and a sharing of expertise among the team members that the child, rather than the individual team members or their professional responsibilities, becomes the most important focus of the team.

The pediatrician and the orthopedist may be joined by other specialists as the need for services arise: neurologists, endocrinologists, cardiologists, and others. Whereas it may seem relatively obvious that these specialities would be considered when the need is apparent, there is one speciality that is often ignored and infrequently included as a part of the total health care of the child with a disability: dental care (Nowak, 1976). "It is the one health problem that affects all handicapped citizens to a degree that has been referred to as catastrophic by many in the health planning profession" (p. 3). There may be several causes for this near or real neglect, including an apathy within the dental and medical professions for dental training and treatment of the child with a disability. Furthermore the parents may view this additional consequence of disability as one more burden to be borne or one more problem to be solved. The often overwhelming requirements of physical and educational care of the child with a disability may be so awesome that the dental care of the child may take a backseat in priorities established by the professionals and the parents alike. Professional and parental education must be provided to help in the establishment of adequate dental hygiene and care for these children.

OCCUPATIONAL AND PHYSICAL THERAPY
Occupational therapy

Occupational therapy has been defined and described in many ways, depending on the type of treatment being used, the type of patient being treated, and the type of disability that the patient may have. A definition that has recently been adopted provides a statement of the range of activity in this health profession:

> Occupational therapy is the application of occupation, any activity in which one engages for evaluation, diagnosis, and treatment of problems interfering with functional performance in persons impaired by physical illness or injury, emotional disorder, congenital or developmental disability, or the aging process in order to achieve optimum functioning, and for prevention and health maintenance. Specific occupational therapy services include, but are not limited to, activities of daily living (ADL); the design, fabrication, and application of splints; sensorimotor activities; the use of specifically designed crafts; guidance in the selection and use of adaptive equipment; therapeutic activities to enhance functional performance; prevocational evaluation and training; and consultation concerning the adaptation of physical environments for the handicapped. These services are provided to individuals or groups through medical, health, educational and social systems, and for the maintenance of health through these systems. (American Occupational Therapy Association, 1977, p. 4)

An expansion of this definition might be useful in light of the range of treatment types possible. The occupational therapist may be involved in (1) assessment of an individual's functional ability both in terms of physical capability and cognitive and/or perceptual abilities; (2) treatment for maintenance of acquired levels of health and physical status; (3) preventive treatment to reduce or limit the effects of a disability and its possible progression; and (4) developmental or redevelopmental treatment to learn new skills and abilities or to relearn skills and abilities that have been lost as a result of illness or injury. The occupational therapist's patients may range in age from early infancy to the geriatric years, and the range of health problems that are referred for treatment is as broad, including failure to thrive; congenital physical disabilities; acquired disabilities through injury, disease, or the aging process; and problems related to psychiatric disorders.

The occupational therapist provides treatment care through the prescription of a physician. The prescription may be to strengthen a specific muscle group, or it may be broader in scope, such as to "develop independent activities of daily living skills."

Treatment of children with physical disabilities may include any of the following activities: perceptual assessment and training to establish the position of the body in space, body image and function, and tactile, kinesthetic, and visual perception (MacDonald, 1970); feeding evaluation and training, including sucking, swallowing, chewing, and tongue thrust problems (Atkins and Chapman, 1975); gross and fine motor activities that might be used in learning finger grasping and release movements required for daily living skills; the development and use of adaptive feeding techniques and of communication equipment such as splints and slings; and the development of skills related to the use of orthotic and prosthetic devices (Willard and Spackman, 1971).

Such activities lead directly to the functioning of the child in the class and should point the way toward a cooperative effort between the occupational therapist and the special education teacher. For example, when the therapist works toward the development of head control in the child with cerebral palsy, the teacher may benefit from this training through the child's ability to better attend to reading activities; when the therapist becomes involved in the development of a special splint or pointing wand or stick for the severely impaired child, the teacher may benefit because of the child's greater potential for communication through the use of a communication board or typewriter (Hunsinger, 1976). Occupational therapy and academic skill development in the classroom need not be mutually exclusive. The cooperation of the professionals in these two areas may result in a program that will meet both the medical and educational needs of the child.

Physical therapy

Physical therapy has, in may ways, problems of definition similar to those found in the field of occupational therapy; the functions and activities of therapy are often related to the type of disability and to the characteristics of the patient. A description of physical therapy and the knowledge that is required of the therapist has been provided by the American Physical Therapy Association:

> Physical therapy requires practical knowledge of human growth and development, human anatomy and physiology, neuroanatomy, neurophysiology, biomechanics of human motion, manifestations of disease and trauma, normal and abnormal psychological responses to injury and disability, and ethnic, cultural and socioeconomic influences on the individual.
>
> The physical therapist practices as a part of a large and varied team of personnel which includes the physician, generally as the team leader, and other professional and assistive health specialists, as well as members of the lay community.(American Physical Therapy Association, 1976)

A distinction that has often been made between occupational and physical therapy has been in the ultimate functioning of the patient: occupational therapy deals with physical functions that enhance daily living activity skills and with the fine and gross motor activities relating to upper-extremity development for the attainment of these skills ; physical therapy deals with physical functions relating to the overall strengthening, positioning, and development of the individual in relation to balance, ambulation, and independent motor functioning.

The treatment process for the child with a physical disability will depend on the nature of the disability, on the physical characteristics of the child, and on the special conditions that may be part of the physician's orders for treatment. Physical therapy, like occupational therapy, is based on the prescription of an attending physician. The prescription may be a request for new information for further treatment (the physician may request an evaluation of muscle strength, range of motion, or other physical characteristics), or the prescription may be for specific treatment. It should include information needed for effective treatment and include diagnosis, treatment goals, the frequency of treatment, the area to be treated, precautions for treatment (information regarding recent surgical procedures, cardiac problems, and so on), and special instructions that the physician may require (for example, exercising with the patient's brace or splint in place) (Downer, 1970). Although the prescription may include a variety of instructions for treatment, the method and type of treatment procedure may be the decision of the therapist involved. The physician may request that the patient develop strength or range of motion of specific muscle groups, but the therapeutic techniques used may be left to the discretion of the therapist. These techniques may include passive or active exercises, stretching, massage, hydrotherapy, electrotherapy, and others.

Another role of both the physical and occupational therapist may be that of consultant or instructor for the child's parents and teacher (Scherzer, Mike, and Ilson, 1976). Because it is often found that the time the child spends in active therapy may be insufficient to reach and maintain the treatment goals established for the child, there may need to be considerable carry-over of therapy to the classroom and the home. For the parent, this may require instruction by the therapist in exercising techniques that will need to be carried out at home; for the teacher, this may require instruction in the posture needs of the child—the child may be required to perform class work in a variety of positions using a variety of therapeutic appliances.

The treatment setting

The organization of therapy centers in schools for the physically disabled has generally been developed around the two therapy classifications; there is usually a physical therapy department or section and an occupational therapy department or section. These departments, headed or supervised by a medical director or chief therapist, have been a part of, and yet apart from, the educational areas. The therapy areas are most frequently located at a site in the school that is separated by some distance from the classroom. In the physical therapy area, equipment such as exercise mats and tables or other devices will be found. The occupational therapy area may have similar equipment but may also have a center where daily living skills may be practiced and developed. The occupational therapy area may include a kitchen, bedroom, and bathroom, in which training in daily living activities may occur, and a shop area with a variety of tools and materials. A treatment and evaluation schedule is arranged between the classroom teacher and the therapists so that children will be released from classroom activities on a regularly scheduled basis (once weekly or once daily, for example) to participate in the treatment program.

Although this may seem to be an appropriate coordination of activities, there is, nevertheless, a separation of functions and a fragmentation of the child's learning that could be avoided. Two changes are beginning to come about in the relationship between therapy and special education for the child with a disability. The distinction between the two separate therapy procedures is becoming less well defined, and the site of treatment is being reconsidered; it is now often found in the classroom rather than in a specific treatment area. The traditional functions and roles of the occupational and physical therapists are becoming more interrelated as such therapists become more involved with the total developmental aspect of treatment. The child is seen as a total entity for care as opposed to the recipient of a collection of treatment procedures and goals. In some instances, this process has reached the level where the identification of the occupational therapist and the physical therapist has given way to that of "medical treatment therapist or specialist," or "developmental therapist." More than a mere name change, however, is apparent. Both types of therapists contribute to the overall evaluation of the child and to the treatment process. The physical, psychosocial, sensory, and educational aspects of physical involvement are being met in the child according to the skills of the therapist rather than according to the traditional professional identification of the therapist.

Both occupational and physical therapy specialists have come to recognize the importance of providing treatment in places other than a clinic setting (MacDonald, 1970; Marx, 1973). Many therapy procedures and techniques may be readily adaptable to the classroom where the child spends the major portion of the school day. This inclusion of therapy in class activities encourages a closer cooperation between therapist and teacher, reduces the amount of time the child spends outside the classroom, provides for follow-up of therapy procedures in the classroom, and reduces the fragmentation of the child between specialists.

The interrelationship of educational and therapeutic goals and interests is evidenced in the evaluation, teaching, and treatment procedures used for a variety of perceptual problems frequently found in children. These problems have long been known as an area of teaching concern because of their impact on learning in the classroom; therapy in relationship to perceptual problems, sensory stimulation, and sensory integration is also well-known and established. Problems in visual perception, figure-ground differentiation, visual-motor coordination, left-right progression, and position in space and body awareness are concerns of equal importance to the teacher (in teaching reading skills) and to the therapist (in developing skills of body control, daily living activities, and other motor functions).

ORTHOPEDIC APPLIANCES

The stigmata often used in identifying children with physical disabilities are those that are most visually obvious: physical abnormalities and mechanical aides used for treatment and/or mobility. Frequently used aides are illustrated in Figs. 4-1 to 4-5. Although these do not cover the full range of appliances that may be seen in any one school, they are representative of those often encountered.

Text continued on p. 76.

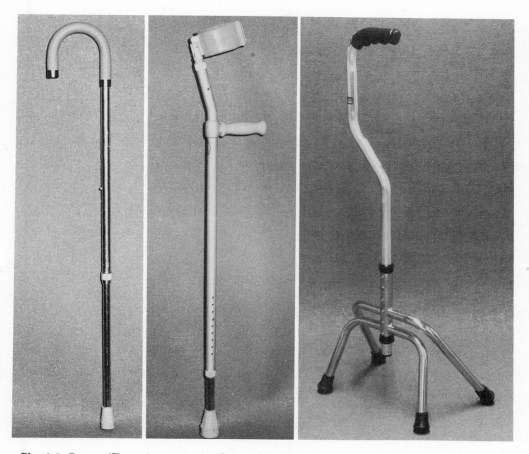

Fig. 4-1. Canes. (From American Academy of Orthopaedic Surgeons. *Atlas of orthotics.* St. Louis: The C. V. Mosby Co., 1975.)

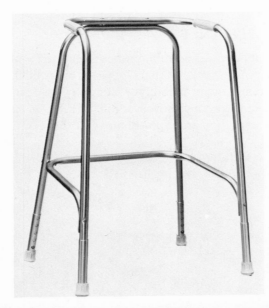

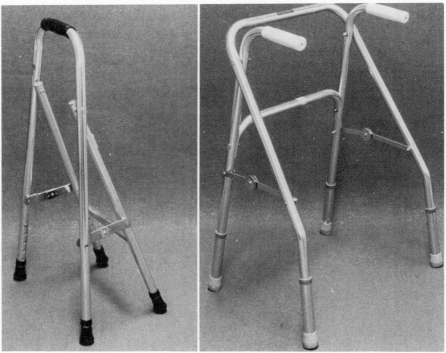

Fig. 4-2. Walkers. (From American Academy of Orthopaedic Surgeons. *Atlas of orthotics.* St. Louis: The C. V. Mosby Co., 1975.)

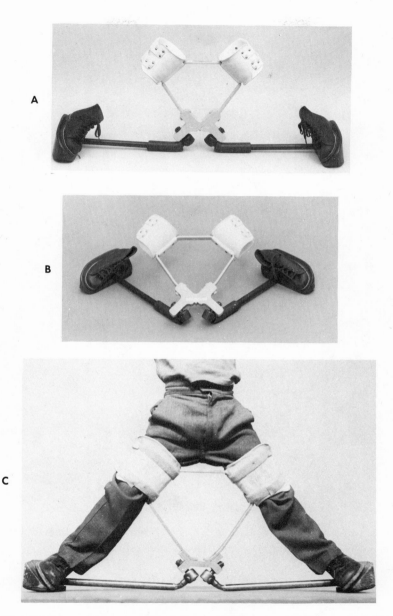

Fig. 4-3. Hip abduction orthosis. **A,** Metal structure and joints; leather or plastic thigh cuffs. Orthosis is jointed, **B,** to allow knee flexion for ambulation, **C,** and sitting while maintaining 45° hip abduction. (From American Academy of Orthopaedic Surgeons. *Atlas of orthotics.* St. Louis: The C. V. Mosby Co., 1975.)

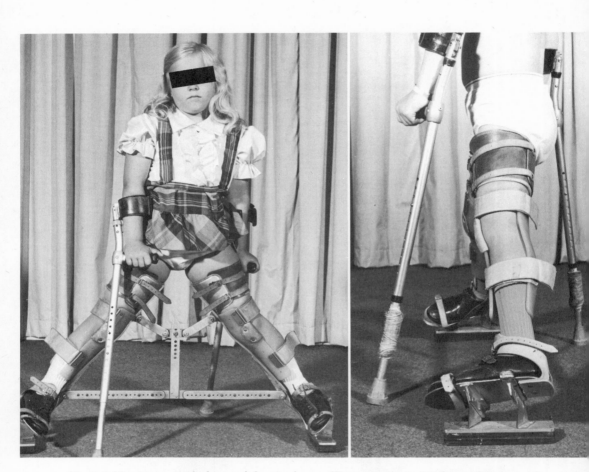

Fig. 4-4. Newington ambulatory abduction brace. (From American Academy of Orthopaedic Surgeons. *Atlas of orthotics*. St. Louis: The C. V. Mosby Co., 1975.)

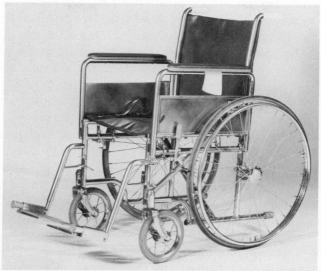

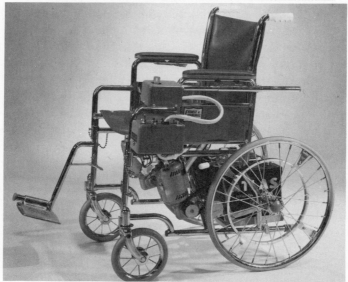

Fig. 4-5. Wheelchairs. (From American Academy of Orthopaedic Surgeons. *Atlas of orthotics*. St. Louis: The C. V. Mosby Co., 1975).

SPEECH/LANGUAGE THERAPY

Of the therapies employed to treat children with physical disabilities, speech therapy is unique in that it is the only therapy responsible for the diagnosis, prescription, and treatment of a specific condition. Although occupational and physical therapy are involved in the evaluation and treatment of the patient, these are done on the prescription of the physician, who is responsible for the diagnosis of the disability. The speech therapist's responsibilities are much broader than those of the other therapy specialists because of this diagnostic role. The range of problems that the speech therapist may deal with is broad, and the problems are complicated not only by their characteristics, but also by their cause.

What does the speech therapist treat? Although the question might better be who does the therapist treat, the answer revolves around the definition of speech problems. How does one define the types of problems that have been referred to the speech therapist? According to Johnson (1967), "A child's speech presents a problem for himself and for others when his listeners pay critical or anxious, or disapproving attention to how he speaks, or are distracted from what he is saying by his way of saying it"(p. 6). This definition is rather general and mechanistic in its approach, however, since the speech therapist must deal with more than the speech production of the child. Consideration must also be given to *language*—the cognitive process whereby meaning and order are associated with sound productions, or words—and to *communication*—the process whereby language is a meaningful exchange between two or more persons.

It is in each of these three areas—speech, language, and communication—that the speech therapist provides service. Children with disabilities vary from those whose speech, language, or communication abilities are within the normal pattern of functioning to those whose physical and mental disabilities exert such an adverse influence that speech is nonintelligible or nonexistent—language is restricted in both its reception and expression, and communication is reduced to a simple binary, yes or no response.

The speech disorders of children with physical disabilities are the same as those that may be found in any other population of children. These include articulation problems (the precision with which words are pronounced according to an identified standard), voice problems (speech characteristics related to the quality of speech sound production), and fluency or rhythm problems (disruptions of speech fluency or rhythm that become a marked characteristic of stuttering).

Articulation problems and voice problems are often of an organic or physical origin; the child may be unable to control the speech and breathing mechanisms to the degree that normal speech or voice production is possible. This may be particularly evident in the child with cerebral palsy; the child may have articulation problems that are directly related to damage to the areas of the brain that control the motor component of speech. This frequently occurring articulation problem, known as dysarthria, "is found in all of those cases of cerebral palsy who have some kind of neuromuscular involvement of the speech mechanism" (Mecham, Berko, and Berko, 1960, p. 72). Other articulation problems may occur because of faulty learning models or as a result of hearing loss (frequently associated with the athetotic type of cerebral palsy). The hearing loss results in a lack of appropriate feedback to the child when he/she begins articulate speech development. Voice problems—those problems that are related to volume, breath control, and pitch—are also often found in children with cerebral palsy. Problems in breath control and the inability to accurately control the speech mechanisms may result in a wide variation of breath, harsh, nasal, and volume characteristics that may add to the problems already mentioned in relation to the articulation of speech sounds. These problems in articulation and voice production, coupled with problems in motor control, and/or drooling, work to depress the frequency and quality of communication effort by those who are so impaired.

In order for communication activities to exist and be fruitful, at least two persons must be active in the process. If one of these two participants in the communication process becomes frustrated in his/her attempts at speech production, or if one of them becomes so distracted and disturbed by the faulty speech attempts of the others, then the communication process breaks down or is terminated. If frustration levels become high enough, communication is not initiated.

In addition to the problems of speech production and communication already mentioned, language processing is of major concern to the speech therapist. Receptive and expressive language may be impaired because of a variety of circumstances, including damage to specific areas of the brain that are related to language processing and the inhibition of the individual from learning the concepts and abstracts of the environment.

The speech therapist's treatment, then, becomes not only one of correcting faulty speech patterns, but also one involving the establishment, and in some cases the reestablishment, of the concepts and conditions needed for effective communication skills. When the child is so severely impaired by a physical disability that communication is not established, and when speech production is nonexistent or unintelligible and an assessment of language is impossible, then other means of communication need to be utilized. The use of binary communication techniques such as yes and no indications by eye blink or another mutually recognized action may be used. This technique is dependent on the finding of a way for the individual to receive and send messages, as well as on the education of others to recognize and use the technique (Moore, 1972).

Another form of communication that has met with considerable success has been the development of "communication boards." These devices, often fitted on the arms of wheelchairs of individuals who have limited or no capabilities for speech provide an opportunity for the child to express thoughts, and communicate with others. Several considerations must be made in the design of such boards: the type and number of words, letters, symbols, or drawings that may be used on the board; the ability of the child to recognize and use the symbols; the structure of the language system; and the physical characteristics of the child in relation to his/her

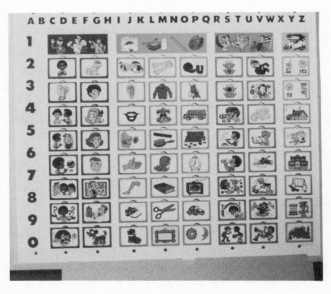

Fig. 4-6. SI/COMM communication board. (Courtesy Carmelita Heiner and SI/COMM.)

needs for communication. The characters that may appear on a board in one situation may be inappropriate in another. Such boards must be flexible in design and must be able to be used and understood by the child, parents, teachers, and others with whom the child has contact (McDonald and Schultz, 1973).

One such board, developed by Heiner (1975), is illustrated in Fig. 4-6. This language board was designed for the child who, though nonverbal, can express ideas to others by pointing to a series of pictures. The pictures, which are color coded, identify personal pronouns, proper nouns, nouns, verbs, and modifiers in a left-to-right progression. This introduction to syntactic structure shows the child that language is ordered and linear. The board may be used in the development of reading readiness skills, as an outlet for communication with others, and as an aid in determining and developing the comprehension of the child. This language board, known as the Si/Comm model, includes a motivation factor whereby the child is encouraged to move beyond the motor limitations imposed by disability so as to extend the possibilities for successful communication.

OTHER PROFESSIONAL SERVICES

Several other professionals are involved in the care, treatment, and welfare of the child with a physical disability and the family. Among those who have particular impact are the social worker and the psychologist. Both of these persons have similar professional concerns as they relate to the child. They often must confront the family and child in times of stress, such as when the impact of disability becomes apparent and intrudes on personal functioning.

Role of the social worker

The social worker may, from the first, be involved with the family when the family must confront the initial crisis: the diagnosis of disability. If the child is born with an obvious physical disability, the social worker may begin interaction with the family in the hospital to help overcome the initial shock of diagnosis confrontation. Expectations for the newly arrived child and expectations that the parents had perceived for themselves in relation to the presence of a normal baby will need resolution. This crisis intervention will continue throughout the growing years of the child when the impact of the effects of the disability on family structure are realized: the requirements of physical care of the growing child; special diets, clothing, and orthopedic appliances that may be required; the role changes that may be imparted to various members of the family; the response to specific characteristics of the disability, such as pain, medical treatment practices, surgery, medication, or financial liability; the different requirements in relation to school experiences that may need to be considered; considerations concerning long-term care and adult life; and the impact of dying and death that may be associated with specific disabilities and illnesses (Travis, 1976).

The stress situations mentioned above are in addition to the specific ones surrounding the individual situation. A different set of circumstances is encountered when the child enters a hospital, receives medical care or treatment, or has been disabled as a result of a painful accident or adult abuse. For example, the child may face the stress of:

> . . . being admitted to the ward or clinic, waiting to hear the diagnosis, frequent change of doctors or nurses, lack of privacy . . . wearing an appliance, taking injections, facing surgery, taking anesthetics, going to bed for a long period, facing a doubtful or poor prognosis, adjusting to a chronic treatment regime . . . (Bartlet, 1961, p. 150)

Feelings of fear, separation, and isolation by the child, and familial attitudes of distrust toward professionals who push and pull at the family's physical, mental, and psychological resources are problems that must be dealt with by the social worker. These client-centered problems are one end of a continuum of concern on the part of the social worker, who must also relate to the various professionals and agencies involved in the treatment and care of the child and the family. Rather than being coordinated in the meeting of needs, the different professionals and agencies may work at odds with one another, even though the aim is to provide the best of comprehensive care. A collaboration of efforts may need to be orchestrated by the social worker, who is in direct contact with all of the principals in the situation. This rather overwhelming task is one that demands knowledge of medical, educational, psychological, and social agency functions and conditions. If there is a possibility for fragmentation of child and family from the various and several persons who propose to serve the child, might not the possibility also exist for the individual members to become fragmented in their own purpose and in their own caring? Caution must be taken to avoid personal and professional dissipation.

Role of the psychologist

The school psychologist is often seen by the teacher as the person who administers intelligence tests and as the culprit behind the involved case descriptions that accompany a child on placement in a class. To be sure, the psychologist *is* responsible for testing and assessment of children and *is* the person responsible for the case studies that accompany children on placement. However, limiting the view of the psychologist to this narrow band of activities does not serve to describe this professional's role. Training in learning theory, in the assessment of learning disabilities, and in the recognition of various learning modalities expands not only the concept of the role, but also of the service area of the school psychologist.

The psychologist is indeed responsible for the administration of a variety of tests to children with a variety of problems, and it is these very problems that make test administration a formidable task. The psychologist must be aware of the types of tests available, their construction, their administration requirements, and their interpretation. For the child with limited motor control, a test that has a motor component must be abandoned or revised. For the child with severe speech and/or language impairment, the psychologist must be aware of the adaptations available for eliciting responses. For the child who is both motorically and speech and/or language impaired, the assessment becomes an even more difficult task. These considerations and others such as the fatigue level of the child, the child's distractibility, and the child's lack of life experiences may tend to depress a measured level of performance and hence not represent a true picture of potential or performance. When dealing with tests involving standardized administration procedures and normed responses, the psychologist must question the use of these tests from the point of view of both actual administration and interpretation (Sattler & Tozier, 1970). The problems associated with test administration are only a few of those directly related to this phase of a school psychologist's function.

Referrals made to the psychologist are often made not only to confirm or identify a particular level of performance of the child, but also because of behaviors exhibited by the child and the parents. Children with physical disabilities may often display signs of stress, tension, distractibility, a dependency on adults fostered by the overprotection of the parents, and anger and striking-out behavior brought on by the frustrations of the disability (Bowley, 1967). These problems, which may reach levels for psychiatric consideration, are often first seen by the psychologist as the child enters specific stages in development: first entry into school; hospital treatments; success or failure in school that may be related to levels of expected accomplishments by the child or the parents; and adolescence, with its attendant problems of reidentification of self, independence seeking, and the need for activity. Although these problems are not unique to the child with a physical disability, it must be recognized that the disability does have an impact on these problems that is unique to the individual and to the life-style imposed on the individual by the disability.

These problems, which are child centered, are in addition to those that may be fostered by, or are a part of, the parents' involvement with the child. All of the problems listed as child centered are, by extension, problems that may be confronting the parents as well. These and problems such as stress from the daily care of the child; financial worries because of the wear and tear of clothes, special diets, or medications; problems with interactions among the family members; and even the inability to get out for an evening's entertainment without worrying about the care of the child are among those that may be presented to the psychologist by the family.

The case study report prepared by the psychologist on the characteristics of the child and the family includes test results, observational data collected during visits with the child and the family, and interpretation of performance in a variety of formal and informal assessment situations. This report becomes a foundation on which recommendations or suggestions may be made for behavior management and remedial techniques designed to stimulate growth and development. The recommendations within these reports may be used at the teacher's discretion and are not mandates for teaching. In consultation with the psychologist, the teacher can, and should, concentrate on the academic skill areas and on the behavioral patterns of the child that will enhance the child's educational and social-emotional growth and development. The ongoing role of the school psychologist as consultant with the teacher and, when needed, with the parents sets into motion the opportunity for continuous assessment and reevaluation of the child's progress. In cooperation with the teacher, this consultant role of the school psychologist has the potential for optimizing the functioning of the child in the school program. It is this interchange of ideas that is the essence of the team approach to serving the child.

Recreational therapy

The goal of services provided by the specialist in recreational therapy is not dissimilar to those provided by the other treatment specialists: participation to the extent possible by the individual in the educational, play, and family activities of the normal population (Frye and Peters, 1972). Many of us, whether disabled or not, need outlets for our nonworking leisure time in order to avoid the stagnation and physical deterioration that results from confinement to the office, business, other work or life setting, or the television set.

Recreational therapy may provide specific therapeutic benefits to those with physical disabilities. These benefits may result in the strengthening of muscles; in perceptual, attitudinal, and self-image improvement; and in the chance to bridge the gap between the sheltered environment of the life of the person with a disability and the community in which recreational opportunities are available (Frye and Peters, 1972; Rathbone and Lucas, 1959). With the increasing availability of public transportation for those with physical disabilities, and even for those who are homebound, the recreational therapist can provide an invaluable service in the training and use of public and private recreational facilities and in the adaptation of games, sports, and other leisure-time pursuits. A person with a disability should not be denied recreational and play activities just because the disability exists. On the other hand, a person with a disability should not be made to feel that participation in any particular activity is a requirement of a recreational setting. Some individuals do prefer passive observation rather than active participation. However, opportunities to learn the skills necessary for participation at whatever level chosen by the individual should be made available to the person with a disability.

Rehabilitation counseling

The role of the rehabilitation counselor and the goal of this professional's services cannot be generalized to the extent that a specific statement about them can be made. The type and severity of disability and the levels of social-emotional-mental development are a part of the rehabilitation and training picture.

> Realistic vocational guidance is indispensable even though it may achieve no more than a healthy psychological and physical state of adjustment. For the great majority, evaluation of assets through intelligence and aptitude testing, prevocational exploratory activities, and workshop evaluation of actual job performance may open brighter perspectives. For some persons a sheltered workshop or homebound activity is desirable, for some further education, and for many competitive employment. (Wright and Trotter, 1968, p. 28)

The role of the vocational rehabilitation counselor not only includes an assessment of the vocational skills of the client and the development of work training and work experience activities, it also involves an active community-based component. Awareness of the community's existing jobs and their requirements, of the job market for the able-bodied and the competition for jobs that this may imply, of the agencies providing services and training for those with disabilities, and of how these community characteristics may be coordinated is an important part of the rehabilitation counselor's function in the placement of clients for both work training and employment.

Teachers, parents, counselors, and others involved with the welfare of children with physical disabilities need to take caution in making assumptions concerning what is to become the adult independence and/or employment status of the child. Physical disability is not a condition for automatic assignment to a sheltered workshop for employment. Work training and work experience, however, are not guarantees of successful employment. Higher education and professional training should not be excluded from consideration for the person with a disability. College graduation and professional training, however, do not place one automatically in the job market. Self-employment need not be excluded from consideration. Persons who are homebound, institution bound, or severely disabled need not necessarily be excluded from employment. Others should not make assumptions or decisions concerning what is or is not appropriate employment or concerning the status that employment choices may have. Usefulness is a part of human dignity, and human dignity may suffer from a lack of usefulness. Employment or work may not be appropriate for everyone. Alternatives should be everyone's right.

SUMMARY

This chapter has reviewed some of the services of professionals involved in the treatment and care of the child with a physical disability and the family. The stress has been on the team approach to the provision of treatment and services. Various physicians have responsibility for the diagnosis and prescription for treatment of disabilities and their accompanying problems and characteristics. Occupational and physical therapists utilize their expertise in devising and implementing treatment modes to carry out these prescriptions for physical management, assessment of functioning, and training in self-care skills. Other ancillary services are provided by speech therapists, social workers, psychologists, recreational therapists, rehabilitation counselors, and others. These professionals bring to the treatment team skills that may be beneficial to the child and the family in making the adjustments necessary for participation in the community.

Despite the possibility of overkill of the notion, the need for cooperation, coordination, communication, and team effort, in its truest sense must be emphasized again and again. Professional status superiority is nonproductive and has the effect of losing sight of the purpose: the child. The only *star* of the team should be the child, and all the players should strive to make it so.

REFERENCES

Atkins, J. A., and Chapman, R. L. Occupational therapy in a myelomeningocele clinic. *American Journal of Occupational Therapy*, 1975, *29*, 403-406.

American Occupational Therapy Association. *Occupational Therapy Newspaper*, 1977, *31* (6):4.

American Physical Therapy Association, Inc. *School of Physical Therapy*. Los Angeles: Childrens Hospital of Los Angeles, 1976.

Bartlett, H. M. *Social work practice in the health field*. New York: National Association of Social Workers, 1961.

Bowley, A. H. A follow-up study of 64 children with cerebral palsy. *Developmental Medicine and Child Neurology*, 1967, *9*, 172-182.

Curtis, B. H. The team approach. In American Academy of Orthopaedic Surgeons, *Symposium on Myelomeningocele*. St. Louis: The C. V. Mosby Co., 1972.

Deaver, G. G. The orthopedically handicapped child. In H. M. Smith (Ed.), *Pediatric problems in clinical practice: special medical and psychological aspects*. New York: Grune & Stratton, Inc., 1954.

Dower, A. H. *Physical therapy procedures: selected techniques*. Springfield, Ill.: Charles C Thomas, Publisher, 1970.

Frye, V., and Peters, M. *Therapeutic recreation: its theory, philosophy, and practice*. Harrisburg, Pa.: Stackpole Books, 1972.

Gottlieb, M. I. Educational health and development. In J. G. Hughes (Ed.), *Synopsis of pediatrics* (4th ed.). St. Louis: The C. V. Mosby Co., 1975.

Heiner, C. *Si/Comm manual: a system of communication for non-verbal children (an experimental model)*. Playa Del Rey, Calif.: Si/Comm, 1975.

Hunsinger, K. W. A simple headstick for cerebral palsied children. *American Journal of Occupational Therapy*, 1976, *30*, 506.

Johnson, W. *Speech handicapped school children* (3rd ed.). New York: Harper & Row, Publishers, Inc., 1967.

Keats, S. *Operative orthopedics in cerebral palsy*. Springfield, Ill.: Charles C Thomas, Publisher, 1970.

MacDonald, E. M. (Ed.). *Occupational therapy in rehabilitation*. London: Bulliere, Tindall and Cassell, 1970.

Marx, M. Integrating physical therapy into a cerebral palsy early education program. *Physical Therapy*, 1973, *53*, 512-514.

McDonald, E. T., and Schultz, A. R. Communication boards for cerebral palsied children. *Journal of Speech and Hearing Disorders,* 1973, *38,* 73-88.

Mecham, M. J., Berko, M. J., and Berko, F. G. *Speech therapy in cerebral palsy.* Springfield, Ill.: Charles C Thomas, Publishers, 1960.

Moore, M. V. Binary communication for the severely handicapped. *Archives of Physical Medicine and Rehabilitation,* 1972, *53,* 532-533.

Nowak, A. J. *Dentistry for the handicapped patient.* St. Louis: The C. V. Mosby Co., 1976.

Rathbone, J. L., and Lucas, C. *Recreation in total rehabilitation.* Springfield, Ill.: Charles C Thomas, Publisher, 1959.

Sattler, J. M., and Tozier, L.L. A review of intelligence test modifications used with cerebral palsied and other handicapped groups. *Journal of Special Education,* 1970, *4,* 391-398.

Scherzer, A. L., Mike, V., and Ilson, J. Physical therapy as a determinant of change in the cerebral palsied infant. *Pediatrics,* 1976, *58,* 47-52.

Travis, G. *Chronic illness in children.* Stanford, Calif.: Stanford University Press, 1976.

Willard, H. S., and Spackman, C. S. *Occupational therapy* (4th ed.). Philadelphia: J. B. Lippincott Co., 1971.

Wright, G. N., and Trotter, A. B. *Rehabilitation research.* Madison, Wisc.: University of Wisconsin, 1968.

LEARNING AND EDUCATIONAL CONCERNS

5 Implications for learning

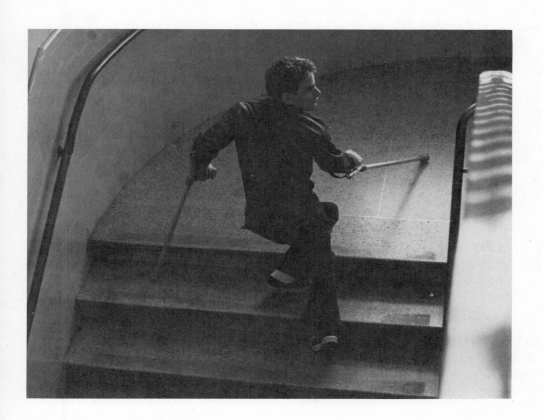

Are there implications for learning because of physical disability? If there are implications, what are they? Are disabilities alike in their implications for learning? What disabilities produce what implications for learning, and what type of learning is implied? These questions might be considered in a perspective of mechanical issues: the impact of body or brain impairment on learning, growth, and development. Another issue that may be considered is not directly related to the mechanical issue but relies on a societal, perhaps philosophical, plane. Have conditions for learning about the society in which persons with physical disabilities live been restricted by that society, so that these individuals have been denied full societal membership with its attendant responsibilities?

In addition to the mechanical differences setting those with physical disabilities apart from others, differences have been perceived that have had an indirect impact on learning and on the availability of learning experiences. An inability to walk impairs the ability of an individual to explore the environment, but the judgment by others that this individual is different from those who can walk is just as limiting to the person's development of concepts that are a part of the environment. Whether the restrictions have a mechanical or physical base, or one that is imposed by society, learning may be impaired as a result of physical disability or limitation.

It has been noted elsewhere that there are several physical disabilities with associated problems that may specifically be identified; cerebral palsy may be accompanied by mental retardation or by various perceptual and/or sensory acuity problems, as may other physical disabilities. Generalizations about these problems are difficult to make in relation to learning, however, since two disability types with the same or highly similar clinical characteristics may not have the same or even remotely similar problems in relation to learning. Each child must be considered individually, not as a part of a clinical grouping; thus, the following discussion of learning problems often found in children with physical disabilities will, of necessity, lack the specificity of a one-to-one relationship; a specific physical characteristic does not necessarily give rise to a specific learning characteristic.

EFFECTS OF DISABILITY ON GROWTH AND DEVELOPMENT
Motor activities

To discuss or consider any of the components of learning—memory, concept formation, or language development—or any of the subcomponents of these characteristics in isolation is unrealistic. Function and development do not occur without an integration of all the component parts. However, there are specific problems in motor development areas that result from impaired mobility. The presence of a physical deviation may produce at least two separate conditions restricting learning: delayed motor development and inaccurate motor functioning. An example of early delayed development is provided by Apgar and Beck (1974) in their contrast of the development of normal infants and infants with cerebral palsy:

Normally . . . an infant learns to lift his head by himself when lying on his stomach sometime between the ages of one and three months. But the average baby with cerebral palsy does not develop this ability until his first birthday. The average normal baby can sit without support by the time he is about eight months old. But the cerebral palsied youngster cannot sit independently until he is about 20 months old. A normal baby crawls by age seven or eight months; a cerebral palsied child at an average age of 26 months. (p. 151)

This delay, which continues throughout the developmental years of the child, may not only result in a lag in the emergence of specific activities and skills, it may also have the effect for the child of reducing the quantity and the quality of experiences available because of the transience of any particular event. In this instance, an opportunity for learning may be denied not because of its nonexistence but because of the nonexistence of the stage of development required for physical control.

The inaccuracy of motor functioning that may be characteristic of the physical deviation is related to the quality of the physical activity generated by the child. Faulty or inaccurate movement may result in an inability to explore environmental conditions requiring specific manipulation for accurate (proper) interpretation. Faulty interpretation of stimuli may result in the establishment of continued altered quality in motor function because of the altered interaction experience, the consequent feedback from interaction, and the incorrect learning of the characteristics of the subject source. If original faulty patterns of movement are repeated, the result is a perpetuation of the faulty movements (Finnie, 1975). This pattern of movement and its consequences for learning are shown diagrammatically in Fig. 5-1.

Motor activities are used constantly in the development and growth of a repertoire of concepts for the child. The child learns the concepts of *up-down, in-out, front-back,* and body and object limits. The child also learns spatial awareness and the differentiation of self and nonself (Whitecroft, 1972). Impairment of this learn-

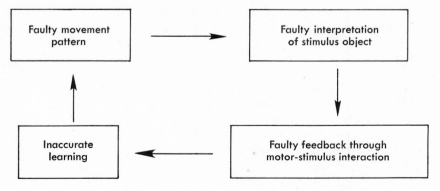

Fig. 5-1. Learning feedback loop in motor activity.

ing may result from the restrictions directly imposed by the physical limitation, from restrictions imposed on the child by overprotective parents (because of fear of the consequences of inaccurate or poor motor control), and from the frustrations of acknowledged poor quality of motor-environment interaction and the consequences of these frustrations. Finally, the total energy requirement may be such that the task is simply not worth the effort.

The implications for the teacher are numerous. Learning deprivation because of motor dysfunction in physical development may require that the teacher not take for granted that motor or physical experiences have occurred, that the concepts that might normally be expected as a result of such experiences have been obtained and utilized, or that the child even knows what to expect or do in relation to his/her own body or motor function and the environmental stimuli confronting the child. In addition, motor activities that also have haptic features (relating to the sense of touch) may affect the child's participation in such school-related activities as block play or writing and/or typing and the child's development of driving and other adult or independent skills.

Visual acuity and perception

The role of vision in learning about the self and the self's interaction with the environment is staggering. To suggest that there is complexity to the visual process is to make an understatement without comparison. Vision is the great organizer of environmental input and as such includes the activities of stimulus reception and perception.

Visual reception dysfunction, often thought of in terms of acuity, is a common problem. "Upwards of 75 percent of all Americans wear or should wear glasses. Nearly all of this loss of function is caused by poor optical properties of the eyes themselves" (Haber, 1974, p. 48). These optical properties include distortion of the eyeball shape, which results in problems of nearsightedness and farsightedness, and distortion of the eye lens or cornea, which produces stigmatism. In addition, eye muscle imbalance may contribute to visual reception problems of poor alignment and result in improper or poor convergence of the eyes.

Such visual problems may be remedied through identification of the observable symptoms by the classroom teacher and referral for opthamological examination and prescription of appropriate corrective lenses, exercises, or surgery. The observable symptoms of which the teacher should be aware include:

1. Frequent rubbing of the eyes.
2. Watering of the eyes with close work.
3. Complaint of eyes aching or paining.
4. Redness and discharge in eyes and along the lids.
5. Holding reading material close to the face.
6. Squinting when reading or looking at the blackboard.
7. Irritability when reading.
8. Dizziness or nausea after much close work.

9. Complaint of headaches with use of the eyes.
10. Closing or covering one eye while reading or concentrating.
11. Excessive blinking, scowling, or facial distortions.
12. One eye that occasionally turns in or out as a result of fatigue or excitement or stays turned constantly.
13. Constant tilting of the head to one side.
14. Pointing at words or losing the place while reading.
15. Undue sensitivity to light. (Swallow, 1976, p. 92)

In addition to a consideration of visual reception and the correction of any identified problems, attention should be given to the role of visual perception and its effects on learning. It is difficult, if not inappropriate, to separate these visual tasks. However, they do have differential qualities; it is somewhat like the difference between what one sees and what one thinks one sees. This visual processing, which includes the "receiving, integrating, and decoding or interpreting of visual stimuli has been commonly referred to as visual perception" (Chalfant and Scheffelin, 1969, p. 21). According to Chalfant and Scheffelin, there are three major components of visual perception: (1) spatial awareness, represented by left-right discrimination, the ability to cross the body midline with the hand, depth perception, the awareness of rotations and reversals, and body-in-space awareness; (2) visual discrimination, represented by prominent feature discrimination, figure-ground differentiation, and visual closure; and (3) object recognition, represented by the identification of the whole from its parts.

Of greatest significance to the classroom teacher is the importance that visual perceptual problems have for school learning. Although it is unrealistic to restrict visual perceptual problems to the association of school learning, it is in this sphere that the teacher has the most influence and responsibility. The child will come to the learning setting with a background of poor learning experiences based on previous interactions with environmental stimuli that have required visual perception for interpretation. Reading and its associated skills—perhaps the most revered of school activities—are the areas that seem to be the most vulnerable to visual perceptual problems. The inability to follow left-to-right progression of letters and words or top-to-bottom progression down a page of print, letter reversals and rotations, and so on, are not uncommon problems associated with reading failure.

Swallow (1976) has identified several types of observable behaviors of which the teacher should be aware in assessing the visual perceptual problems of children. The following outline is an adaptation of Swallow's categorization of these behaviors into four major areas:

A. *Visual reception*: Comprehension of the meaning of what is seen.
   1. Doesn't like to look at picture books or magazines.
   2. Responds better to verbal directions than to visual demonstrations.
   3. Doesn't copy letters or numbers well.
   4. Doesn't see humor in pictures when other children do.

  5. Has difficulty understanding size concepts.

  6. Has difficulty matching pictures, symbols, or letters.

 B. *Visual association*: Comprehension of the relationship of things that are seen.

  1. Doesn't make aesthetic comparisons between things ("this is prettier").

  2. Can't categorize pictures in reading readiness activities.

  3. Isn't interested in demonstrations of or experiences with how things work.

  4. Isn't interested in construction toys and can't create with them.

  5. Doesn't engage in creative ("pretend") play with objects.

  6. Doesn't relate objects or pictures that commonly go together.

 C. *Visual closure*: Identification of an object from incomplete visual information.

  1. Has difficulty understanding letters printed in a different style from the ones used in the book or by the teacher.

  2. Is excessively slow in visual work; studies pictures or words for a long time.

  3. Doesn't get a clue from part of a picture drawn by the teacher.

  4. Doesn't understand dot-to-dot drawing.

  5. Doesn't get meaning from sketches or pictures with stick figures.

  6. Doesn't see things unless they are fully exposed (can't find a partially hidden coat in a pile of coats).

 D. *Visual sequencing*: Recognition and/or recall of ordered visual stimuli.

  1. Doesn't wait for his turn in sequential games.

  2. Doesn't recall sequence of landmarks of a familiar route (trip from school bus–loading ramp to the classroom).

  3. Has difficulty learning sight vocabulary words.

  4. Doesn't recognize when something is done out of the usual sequence.

  5. When copying a word, copies one letter at a time and constantly refers back to the word being copied.

  6. Can't sequentially reproduce actions demonstrated by the teacher.

It must be understood that no one, two, or three of the above difficulties are sufficient to identify a child as having a visual perceptual problem. This is not to say that the presence of one or a few of these problems is not meaningful or important; it simply may not be associated with a problem of visual perception, and the teacher should avoid any such categorization or identification. Children frequently do not have all of the skills cited above on entry into school. And frequently children do not learn these skills on the first attempt. However, when the child is consistently deficient in several of these behaviors, the teacher should make every effort to determine precisely the nature of the problem and initiate activities that will be remediative.

Auditory acuity and perception

Hearing, like vision, may be thought of in two contexts: the measurable aspect of the ability to hear and the complex refinements of sound recognition. In the previous section, vision is described as an organizer of the environment for learning; in the same sense, hearing plays a major role in the development of the human characteristic that separates human beings from all other animals: the exchange of ideas through verbal language. The role of hearing in language development, production, and usage, however, is not the only role that hearing plays in our lives. To assess the importance of hearing for yourself, set aside this book for a moment and recall all of the instances during the day when you used your ability to hear, recognize, and discriminate sounds *not directly related to language*. You may have started the day by using your ability to hear in order to wake up—through the noise of the alarm clock. This process, however, is more involved than just hearing the alarm; it includes distinguishing the alarm sound from other noises. This morning, you were able to direct your attention to the source of the sound and locate it in order to turn the alarm off. And so it goes throughout the day—you engage in hearing and processing activities both related and unrelated to language.

An impairment of the ability to hear will have an impact on the processing of the auditory stimuli for appropriate usage. The following are some of the behavioral signs of hearing difficulty; the classroom teacher who identifies these behaviors in a child should refer the child to the school nurse for careful testing (Watkins, 1976):

1. Fails to pay attention when spoken to.
2. Gives wrong answers to simple questions.
3. Often asks the speaker to repeat words or sentences.
4. Has frequent colds and earaches.
5. Fails to articulate certain sounds correctly or omits certain consonant sounds.
6. Is withdrawn and does not mingle readily with classmates.
7. Pays extra attention to the face of the speaker.

If a child's hearing ability is intact and the sound stimuli is not blocked but auditory problems still seem to be present, one must consider the possibility of problems in the processing of sounds. As might be expected, auditory perception is not a single activity but one of a multiplicity of activities or components. The literature is not in agreement as to what constitutes these components or as to how many of them exist. Lerner's (1976) review of the literature has identified several components. Her listing of the specific auditory functions in perception include auditory discrimination, auditory memory, auditory sequencing, and auditory blending. Others have identified additional types of auditory processing activities (Chalfant and Scheffelin, 1969; Swallow, 1976). Making a composite of the lists of auditory perception components seems like a logical procedure but is difficult to do because of a lack of a common vocabulary and set of meanings for terms. The list on p. 94 is offered for consideration.

1. Auditory attending or reception
2. Auditory discrimination
3. Auditory sequencing or memory
4. Auditory figure-ground discrimination

A fifth component is related to the perception of specific aspects of verbal language, including sound blending, closure, and grammatical structure. The following outline is an adaptation of Swallow's observable classroom behaviors for the components listed above:

A. *Auditory attending or reception*: Awareness and understanding of language.
   1. Doesn't correctly answer comprehension questions about a story that has just been read to him/her.
   2. Doesn't laugh at funny stories, nonsense rhymes, or silly language when other children usually do.
   3. Isn't interested in hearing a story read from a book, but likes to look at accompanying pictures.
   4. Doesn't listen to other children recite in "show and tell" or participate in other classroom verbal activities.
   5. Has difficulty understanding what he/she hears on a phonograph, radio, or tape recorder.
B. *Auditory discrimination*: Ability to determine differences between sounds.
   1. Has difficulty discriminating sounds or single speech sounds, or confuses similar sounds (*pin* for *pen*).
   2. Can't identify sounds sources.
   3. Often makes sound substitutions in reading.
   4. May have a problem in articulation.
   5. Has difficulty identifying initial sounds for words in phonics activities.
C. *Auditory sequencing or memory*: Storage and recall of what is heard and the order in which it is heard.
   1. Can't count to ten or recite the alphabet.
   2. Is poor in recalling the oral spelling of a simple word.
   3. Has difficulty recalling a poem, song, or rhyme.
   4. Can't follow a set of directions in correct order ("stand up, get your coat, and go stand by the door").
   5. Can't recall events of the previous day or week in the correct order.
D. *Auditory figure-ground discrimination*: Ability to identify sound within background noise.
   1. Is unable to attend auditorally to speech sounds.
   2. Is easily distracted by sudden background noises or can't work in a noisy room.

3. Can't adjust to a noisy background (children playing in the play yard).
4. When distracted by sound, can't get back to the original task; has a seemingly short attention span.
5. Has more difficulty understanding orally when the teacher moves around the room.

No one or more of these behaviors necessarily implies problems of auditory perception. The key to utilizing these behaviors in the assessment of the presence of a problem is in the consistency with which these problems are presented. Consistency and repetition of these behaviors should give rise to corrective measures by the teacher.

• • •

Why do we need to attend to the motor, visual, and hearing problems of children with physical disabilities? Because they are present, and because they do have an impact on learning. This is one of those times when the most appropriate response to a question is simply "Because!" Because, if we make assumptions about a child's motor or sensory functioning, that assumption can be detrimental to the child's learning and eventual independence. Because, if we don't attend to these problems, the teaching of these children is burdensome without reason or cause. Because, if we can accurately assess the functioning of children in these areas, problems discovered can be attended to and remediation attempted. Because, for the teacher to do less would signify incompetence, irresponsibility, and neglect.

OVERVIEW OF SOME DEVELOPMENTAL THEORIES

Although this book has, as a matter of course, avoided topics with a theoretical base, a complete avoidance of the theories and hypotheses of learning that have been postulated in the field does not seem warranted. Presented here is a brief overview of five theorist-educators and their contributions to education, growth, and development: Jean Piaget (a developmental approach for concept formation), Newell Kephart (the concept of motor learning as a base for development), Bryant Cratty (the concept of movement as an adjunct to learning), and Carl Delacato and Glenn Doman (the concept of neurological organization as a basis for treatment). These five are reviewed here because of the implications of their contributions to the learning of individuals with physical disabilities. The literature on learning, growth, and development is vast. The reader who is interested in developing his/her background in this area is encouraged to review the plentiful resources available.

Jean Piaget

There are few, if any, theorists whose work has generated more thought and research in recent years than that of Piaget. This person has presented order to process and structure to functioning. According to Piaget (1968), mental development occurs during specific stages or periods, and each stage builds or develops on the conditions of the previous stage. These periods and their several subparts, though associated with specific chronological ages, might be better thought of in terms of an identification of the child's general age status. Piaget's developmental periods include:

Age status	Developmental period	Characteristics
Infancy (birth to 2 years, approximately)	Sensorimotor (two previous stages may be included: reflex stage and organization of percepts and habits)	Instinctual events, such as the sucking reflex; the exercise, organization, and coordination of motor and perceptual acts; initial affective organization
Early childhood (2 to 7 years, approximately)	Preoperational thought	Thought development, language usage, use of symbol systems, and intuitional interpersonal feelings
Middle childhood (7 to 12 years, approximately)	Concrete operations	Beginnings of logical thought, and moral and social feelings of cooperation
Adolescence to adulthood (12 years and onward)	Formal operations	More advanced abstract reasoning and logical thought; personality development and social consciousness

Major learning events are acquired through the processes of "assimilation" and "accommodation." Assimilation requires that the

> . . .individual takes within himself certain aspects of the environment and these become organized within classes or groups. . . . In the course of the process, the child is also making adjustments to these new assimilations. This is referred to as accommodation. The child's intellectual development proceeds by the assimilation of new information; this, in turn, results in modification of some existent schema (accommodation). (Sigel, 1975, p. 77)

Piaget's stages of development have had most reference to growth and development in children who are within the normal range of physical and mental characteristics. Little research and application has been directed to populations of children with disabilities (Suppes, 1974). However, Tessier's (1969) work with cerebral-palsied infants has had important implications for the identification of Piagetian stages of development in children with physical disabilities. Tessier found that "very seriously disabled children" do follow Piaget's sensorimotor stage of development. Her findings included not only the presence of the sensorimotor stage, but also a qualitative difference of performance within this period when infants with cerebral palsy were compared to normal infants.

> The CP [cerebral palsy] sample, by comparison to the normal sample, exhibited: slower rate of response to problems; need for more trials in problem solving tasks; more limited range of interactions with objects and toys; lower level of frustration tolerance; and the need for more encouragement from the examiner to attend to tasks at hand. (Tessier, 1969, pp. 93-94)

Furth's (1970) suggestion that Piaget's theory of development should have its first application in early childhood education programs is supported by Tessier, who sees a "need for incorporating more intense and extensive sensorimotor activities and experiences into therapeutic programs in the early years" (pp. 94-95).

Newell Kephart

The infant's first learning is of a muscular and motor nature. It is from this premise that Kephart (1960) theorizes that "to a large extent, so-called higher forms of behavior develop out of and have their roots in motor learning" (p. 35).

As children develop from their initial motor experiences, other functions are also being exercised. Sensory-perceptual activities, which develop in conjunction and in coordination with motor activities, help "the child establish a solid and reliable concept of the world" (Lerner, 1976, p. 142).

The motor bases of the perceptual-motor process are of particular importance to those concerned with children with physical disabilities. Motor generalizations are developed from a series of motor patterns known by the child to have a specific purpose or function. Three of these motor generalizations are thought to be of particular importance to education: balance and posture, locomotion, and contact, receipt and propulsion (Chaney and Kephart, 1968).

Balance and posture are experienced by the child in relation to a universal environmental condition: gravity. The states of balance and posture help to establish the child's awareness of body position in relation to all other environmental objects. This awareness is a part of spatial relationships, which become important in the active exploration of the environment. The importance that Kephart attaches to posture can be seen in his statement that "all movement patterns, and consequently all behavior, must develop out of the posturing mechanisms. Movement not in accord with basic posture cannot be performed" (Chaney and Kephart, 1968, pp. 39-40).

Locomotion for the child is quite simply the movement of the body through space and the relationship of the body with other objects as the child moves or as the objects move. The activities of crawling, walking, and running, as well as all other movement activities, help the child establish a knowledge of the relationship between the body and objects in space.

The third motor generalization is that of contact, receipt and propulsion. Contact is that means by which the child explores the objects in his/her world and discovers their characteristics. The three elements of contact as defined by Kephart are reaching, grasping, and releasing. Primarily functions of the hand, these activities require the child to extend him/herself for contact and attach and detach him/herself. These manipulatory functions form the basis for a large part of the explorations of the growing child. Receipt and propulsion relate to body functioning as objects in the environment move toward and away from the body. Stopping and catching moving objects and pushing or throwing are examples of receipt and propulsion.

For children with physical disabilities resulting in impaired posture and balance, locomotion, and the activities of contact, receipt and propulsion, the quality of learning experiences will be diminished. The child's limited physical capacity for movement and exploration may be further limited by concerns of the parents for the child's safety and protection. These parental concerns, though real, add another dimension to the deprivation of learning and its consequences for school-related activities.

Bryant J. Cratty

Cratty (1969 b) "does not feel that movement is the basis of the intellect" (pp. 1-2). This single statement probably is the most distinguishing feature of Cratty's position toward learning. According to Cratty (1967), although movement is an important dimension in human behavior, its importance lies in its potential for numerous educational activities. In addition to the benefits derived from the self-satisfaction of being able to perform motor activities, the child is also able to enhance his/her self-image and peer acceptance through individual activities and group play.

Cratty has developed a variety of organized movement activities and games that are useful in extending attention to task, perceptual development, language and number skills, and other school-related achievements. According to Cratty (1969 b), there are several reasons for employing movement activities in education: (1) the child is provided a means for acting out his/her thought processes; (2) simple responses to various stimuli may be made; (3) movement activities are fun and motivating; (4) movement activities may be used as a methodology when other techniques have failed; (5) motor tasks may involve both movement and perceptual skills; and (6) movement has qualities of the "here" and "now," of the obvious rather than the subtle.

In addition to general movement activities, Cratty has made several suggestions for the development of games and activities for children with physical disabilities (Cratty, 1969a; Cratty and Breen, 1972). Participation in games and motor activities by children with disabilities may be very successful if these are at an appropriate physical level. On the other hand, if such children experience failure in participation, it may be detrimental to their self-concept and feelings about their disability (Cratty and Breen, 1972). Every effort needs to be made to analyze the capabilities of the child in order to plan and implement activities that will have as high a degree of success probability as possible. Cratty (1969a) has suggested several cautions to be taken in developing physical activities for children with physical disabilities:

1. Consult the recommendations of the child's physician for the level of physical involvement that is safe for a specific child.
2. Carefully monitor the vigor and duration of the game or activity so as to avoid physical exertion of the child.

3. Avoid excess competition. Past failures may not have developed in the child a sense of sportsmanship or striving for successful participation.
4. Be aware that a game or activity in which a child is excessively motivated may cause the child to move more rapidly and/or with less judgment than otherwise.
5. Be aware that game rules may be confusing and not clearly understood by the child because of a lack of previous experience in organized activities.

Carl Delacato and Glenn Doman

Carl Delacato and Glenn Doman, founders of the Institute for the Achievement of Human Potential, have developed a concept of neurological organization that has been the basis for their treatment of children with reading, mobility, and perceptual problems. This organizational theory suggests that neurological development proceeds up the spinal cord through the medulla, pons, and midbrain, ending at the cortex level. Development at each of these levels has specific functions that are reportedly associated with the functions of mobility, language, vision, hearing, and touch. The highest level of development is the establishment of hemisphere dominance. A failure to develop according to this scheme results in problems in mobility or communication.

> Those areas of neurological organization which have not been completed or are absent are overcome by *passively imposing* them upon the nervous system in those problems of mobility and are taught to those with problems of speech or reading. When the neurological organization is complete the problem is overcome. (Delacato, 1963, p. 7)

Treatment for these problems is often placed in the hands of the parents, who are taught to perform a variety of activities with the child, depending on the child's level of neurological organization and hence on the level of intervention needed. Treatment has been reported to fall into two categories: crawling and creeping, and patterning.

> The children are patterned for five minutes, four times daily, seven days a week without exception. The patterns are administered by three adults. One adult turns the head, another moves the right arm and leg, and the third moves the left arm and leg. (Delacato, 1963, p. 72)

Claims of success through this treatment process based on the theory of neurological organization have come under attack and scrutiny in both the popular (Newsweek, 11/13/67; Time, 5/31/68) and professional literature (Cruickshank, 1968; Freeman, 1967; Glass and Robbins, 1967; Robbins, 1966). In their review of the literature cited by Delacato as support of the theory and procedural successes Glass and Robbins state that "without exception, these experiments contained major faults in design and analysis" (p. 49) and put into question the validity of the reference as support. In a study to test the theoretical and practical implications of the theory of neurological organization, Robbins found that "since the central concept of the theory—the relationship between neurological organization and reading—has not been supported by the findings, the entire theory is suspect" (p. 523).

Although Lerner (1976) has stated that many parents support the theory and its related techniques, the professional community has published opposition statements calling into question the neurological theory and the lack of data to support claimed treatment successes. It is interesting to compare Lerner's statement regarding parents with the concerns expressed in the *Archives of Physical Medicine and Rehabilitation* in this journal's (1968) official statement regarding the Doman-Delacato treatment: "The regimens prescribed are so demanding and inflexible that they may lead to neglect of other family members' needs"(p. 183).

THE TEACHER OF CHILDREN WITH PHYSICAL DISABILITIES

Thus far in this book, a myriad of facts, implications, and suppositions regarding the characteristics and nature of children with physical disabilities has been presented. Attention now is directed toward the teacher who is responsible for the education and training of these children. What are the characteristics of this teacher? What type of training must be provided for this person to be able to meet the needs of the children for whom he/she will have ultimate responsibility? What components of a training program are necessary and in what order, for adequate teacher preparation? These and several thousand other questions can be asked and answered according to the individual teacher's needs, the needs of the children involved, and the needs or imposed requirements of the community and society.

In an effort to identify successful teachers of children with mental and physical disabilities, Meisgeier (1965) has provided an almost overwhelming list of desirable characteristics. A listing of these personal qualities includes high intelligence; a good attitude toward children and teaching; high achievement in college preparation courses; an adventurous, experimenting and impulsive nature; readiness to try new ideas; responsiveness; friendliness; cheerfulness; sociability; the ability to remain unannoyed at leaving a task unfinished; an even disposition; the ability to remain calm in a crisis; the ability to face emotional situations without fatigue; emotional stability; freedom from nervous and instability symptoms; a vigorous, energetic, enthusiastic, talkative, and expressive personality; alertness; extroversion; responsibility; independence; leadership ability to organize, promote new projects, and influence others; and the ability to be realistic, practical, and logical.

The only qualities or characteristics of life that seem to be left out are those indicated in the Boy Scout and Girl Scout oathes, the Ten Commandments, and the Golden Rule! Are there any of us who qualify?

In addition to the above personal qualities, Wyatt (1970) has listed a variety of specific teaching skills at least as complex as the disabilities of the children: Included are those of:

1. Diagnostic and assessment skills;
2. A functional, medical, and therapeutic vocabulary;
3. An appreciation of the roles of specialists who work in the other disciplines;
4. An advanced knowledge of educational technology;
5. A sound understanding of all areas of exceptionality;
6. The ability to integrate academic learning with the objectives of vocational education and rehabilitation;
7. The ability to provide counseling to students and their parents;
8. Familiarity with the other social agencies relating to the students;
9. The ability to effectively interpret both the program and students' needs to professional colleagues;
10. An ability to absorb research and translate it into educational practice;
11. A willingness to objectively assess the success of the program and to modify it as necessary;
12. Capacity to maintain personal equilibrium. (p. 41)

Teacher preparation

In the teaching as well as in the preparation of teachers of children with physical disabilities one needs to ask what is significantly different about these children to require special techniques and training. The first and most obvious response to this question is the presence of physical disability. The next response probably concerns the impact that disability has on learning. A large proportion of the population of school-aged children with physical disabilities is now being served in regular education classes with able-bodied peers, or soon will be. For this group, neither the physical limitations imposed by disability nor the impact of disability on learning prohibits the children from participating in what might be termed a traditional educational setting. What is left for consideration, then, is the population of children who "manifest multi-sensory deficiencies, perceptual inadequacies, communication barriers, social and emotional complexities, and retarded intellectual ability" (Wald, 1970, p. 95). Because of the nature of these disabilities, which occur in addition to physical limitations, it is proposed here that the child with multiple disabilities be considered from the perspective of the learning disability model rather than from the traditional perspective of the medical model. The learning disability model for intervention, as opposed to the medical model, directs attention to the impact of the physical limitation on learning, rather than suggesting that the physical limitation itself is the educational problem.

The elements that should constitute a teacher-training program are as varied as the programs and the institutions in which they are provided. A national leadership document on the preparation of teachers of children with physical disabilities has outlined five basic elements that teacher-training programs should include: (1) prescreening and counseling of candidates; (2) interaction with the total university; (3) interaction with community representatives, other institutions, and agencies; (4) use of program components of practicum, curriculum, and methods of instruction; and (5) commitment to certain ethical positions (competency-based instruction and teacher-educator's accountability) (Bigge, 1973, p. 18).

A teacher-training program that encompasses each of the above elements plus those mandated by the state government is presented below. This training program, which was developed using a learning disability model, requires the following as a prerequisite: a bachelor of arts degree in an acceptable major, a minimum grade point average, and certification to teach "normal" children (such certification may be acquired concurrently with a specialist credential). This competency-based training program requires a generic program of preparation for all teacher candidates as well as training in a specific disability area. Four areas for which demonstrable competencies are required include *pupil assessment, instruction, evaluation of pupil progress and program effectiveness,* and *professional interpersonal relationships.* The program presented here is an adaptation of the one developed by the Department of Special Education, School of Education, California State University, Los Angeles, (1974). In the interests of space, the program presented here is not in a specific competency statement format; rather competency area requirements are stated.

Competency-based Training Program

Prior to entrance into the applied portion of the basic generic program, candidates are required to complete an introductory sequence encompassing two sets of competencies: (1) knowledge of the physical, cognitive, social, and personality development of the normal child from gestation through adolescence and (2) knowledge of the types, nature, and extent of the various categories of exceptionalities of individuals; state and federal laws and provisions related to exceptional children and adults; types of educational programs for the various exceptionalities; the current state of the art in teaching exceptional individuals; and current issues and trends in educating exceptional individuals.

A. The basic generic program shall provide for the development of understandings and demonstrable competencies in pupil assessment. Candidates are expected to be able to demonstrate competence in each of the following areas:

1. Recognition of behavioral commonalities among exceptional students.

2. Utilization of current principles, procedures, techniques, and instrumentation in assessing learning and behavioral patterns in exceptional students.

3. Assessment of the characteristics and behavior of exceptional students in terms of program and development needs.

B. The basic generic program shall provide for the development of understandings and demonstrable competencies in the instruction of special education students. Candidates are expected to be able to demonstrate competence in each of the following areas:

1. Development and effective use of individualized behavioral and instructional objectives.
2. Development and effective use of appropriate individualized instructional processes and strategies.

C. The basic program shall provide for the development of understandings and demonstrable competencies in the evaluation of student progress and program effectiveness. Candidates are expected to be able to demonstrate competence in each of the following areas:
   1. Designing and utilization of student performance criteria to evaluate student learning and behavior.
   2. Evaluation and reporting of outcomes of a teacher-learning sequence to students and parents and for school records in terms of stated objectives.
   3. Evaluation of teaching methods, materials, and media in terms of efficiency in attaining stated objectives.

D. The basic program shall provide for the development of understandings and demonstrable competencies in professional interpersonal relationships. Candidates are expected to be able to demonstrate competence in each of the following areas:
   1. Utilization of management, communication, and supervisory skills to implement effectively the educational process among administrators, teachers, aides, service personnel, and students.
   2. Utilization and implementation of self-assessment techniques for the improvement and development of self-concept and open communication techniques.

E. Preparation for specialization in the physical disability area shall provide for the development of understandings and demonstrable competencies in the assessment of students with physical disabilities. Candidates are expected to be able to demonstrate competence in each of the following areas:
   1. Assessment of physical, intellectual, social, and emotional characteristics of both physically disabled and nondisabled students.
   2. Assessment of learning disabilities in relation to psychological, genetic, physiological, social, and cultural conditions.
   3. Assessment of motivational and attitudinal differences, including, but not limited to, self-control, anxiety, general attitudes toward learning, and the acceptance of success.
   4. Utilization of systematic observation, academic assessment, clinical teaching, and specialized formal assessment procedures for individualized instruction.
   5. Assessment of specific implications of physical disabilities in relation to learning and maturational growth sequences, including career preparation, in the instructional program.

F. Preparation for specialization in the physical disability area shall provide for the development of understandings and demonstrable competencies in the instruction of students with physical disabilities. Candidates are expected to be able to demonstrate competence in each of the following areas:

1. Identification of current issues and trends and utilization of research findings in program implementation.
2. Counseling of students with physical disabilities and their parents.
3. Identification, development, and utilization of appropriate materials modification, innovative teaching strategies, new orthopedic appliances or other prosthetic equipment, and innovative modifications of the classroom environment to accommodate the students with physical disabilities.

G. Preparation for specialization in the physical disability area shall provide for the development of understandings and demonstrable competencies in the evaluation of the progress of students with physical disabilities and in the evaluation of program effectiveness. Candidates are expected to be able to demonstrate competence in each of the following areas:

1. Description and evaluation of several theoretical instructional systems used with students with physical disabilities.
2. Analysis and evaluation of all program elements unique to an educational setting for students with physical disabilities.

H. Preparation for specialization in the physical disability area shall provide for the development of understandings and demonstrable competencies in professional interpersonal relationships. Candidates are expected to be able to demonstrate competence in each of the following areas:

1. Application of appropriate intervention techniques to extend the personal interactions of students with their peers and adults.
2. Planning and conducting parent meetings to discuss program objectives and procedures in an educational setting for students with physical disabilities.
3. Utilization of ethical practices in communication to others about individual student characteristics, problems, and needs.
4. Initiation and pursuit of a program of self-assessment and professional improvement.

SUMMARY

The problems associated with impaired motor functioning, and with visual and auditory acuity and perception have been discussed in relation to their impact on learning for children with physical disabilities. The implications of specific characteristics or sets of characteristics for learning can be readily seen as these relate to the many physical limitations found in such children. Learning theorists and their contributions to an understanding of the growth and development of children with physical disabilities have also been reviewed. Although not an all-inclusive presentation of the implications of physical disability for learning, this chapter should provide some insight into the impact that the one has on the other.

The final section of the chapter deals with the teacher of children with physical disabilities. Who is this person, and what competencies and skills are needed for the teacher to be effective? In trying to answer these questions, one should not be overwhelmed by either the requirements or the rewards. Those who enter this unique teaching field will find and develop the skills and competencies needed by and demanded of both the children and the profession.

No one ever said it was going to be easy. But it is fun, and it is rewarding.

REFERENCES

Apgar, V., and Beck, J. *Is my baby all right?* New York: Simon & Schuster, Inc., 1974.

Archives of Physical Medicine and Rehabilitation. Official statement—the Doman-Delacato treatment of neurologically handicapped children. *Archives of Physical Medicine and Rehabilitation*, 1968, *49*, 183-186.

Bigge, J. Teacher education for COHI-MH. In F. P. Connor and M. Cohen (Eds.), *Leadership preparation for educators of crippled and other health impaired-multiply handicapped populations; proceedings of a special study institute, Tappen Zee Inn, Nyack, New York, March 28-31, 1973.* New York: Teachers College Press, 1973.

Chalfant, J. C., and Scheffelin, M. A. *Central processing dysfunctions in children: a review of research.* National Institute of Neurological Diseases and Stroke (NINDS) Monograph No. 9. Washington, D.C.: Department of Health, Education, and Welfare, 1969.

Chaney, C. N., and Kephart, N. C. *Motoric aids to perceptual training.* Columbus, Ohio: Charles E. Merrill Publishing Co., 1968.

Cratty, B. J. *Movement behavior and motor learning* (2nd ed.). Philadelphia: Lea & Febiger, 1967.

Cratty, B. J. *Developmental games for physically handicapped children.* Palo Alto, Calif: Peek Publications, 1969. (a)

Cratty, B. J. *Movement, perception and thought: the use of total body movement as a learning modality.* Palo Alto, Calif.: Peek Publications, 1969. (b)

Cratty, B. J., and Breen, J. E. *Educational games for physically handicapped children.* Denver: Love Publishing Co., 1972.

Cruickshank, W. M. To the editor. *Exceptional Children*, 1968, *35*, 93-94.

Delacato, C. H. *The diagnosis and treatment of speech and reading problems.* Springfield, Ill.: Charles C Thomas, Publisher, 1963.

Department of Special Education, School of Education, California State University, Los Angeles. *Professional preparation program plan for the specialist credential in communication handicapped, physically handicapped, learning handicapped, severely handicapped, gifted.* Los Angeles: The Department, 1974.

Finnie, N. R. *Handling the young cerebral palsied child at home* (2nd ed.). New York, E. P. Dutton and Co., Inc. 1975.

Freeman, R. D. Controversy over "patterning" as a treatment for brain damage in children. *Journal of the American Medical Association*, 1967, *202*, 385-388.

Furth, H. G. *Piaget for teachers.* Englewood Cliffs, N.J.: Prentice-Hall, Inc., 1970.

Glass, G. V., and Robbins, M. P. A critique of experiments on the role of neurological organization in reading performance. *Reading Research Quarterly*, 1967, *3*, 5-51.

Haber, R. N. Visual perception. In Department of Health, Education, and Welfare, *Psychology and the handicapped child.* Publication No. (OE) 73-05000. Washington, D.C.: The Department, 1974.

Kephart, N. C. *The slow learner in the classroom.* Columbus, Ohio: Charles E. Merrill Publishing Co., 1960.

Lerner, J. W. *Children with learning disabilities* (2nd ed.). Boston: Houghton Mifflin Co., 1976.

Meisgeier, C. The identification of successful teachers of mentally or physically handicapped children. *Exceptional Children*, 1965, *32*, 229-235.

Piaget, J. *Six psychological studies.* New York: Alfred A. Knopf, Inc., 1968.

Robbins, M. P. A study of the validity of Delacato's theory of neurological organization. *Exceptional Children*, 1966, *32*, 517-523.

Sigel, I. Concept formation. In J. J. Gallagher (Ed.), *The application of child research to exceptional children.* Reston, Va.: The Council for Exceptional Children, 1975.

Suppes, P. Cognition: a survey. In Department of Health, Education, and Welfare, *Psychology and the handicapped child.* Publication No. (OE) 73-05000. Washington, D.C.: The Department, 1974.

Swallow, R. Observable symptoms of visual difficulty; behavioral signs: possible hearing disorders. In A. V. Watkins (Ed), *Syllabus for generic core classes.* Los Angeles: Department of

Special Education, California State University, Los Angeles: 1976.

Tessier, F. A. The development of young cerebral palsied children according to Piaget's sensorimotor theory. Unpublished doctoral dissertation, University of California, Los Angeles, 1969.

Wald, J. R. Crippled and other health impaired and their education. In F. P. Connor, J. R. Wald, and M. J. Cohen (Eds), *Professional preparation for educators of crippled children; proceedings of a special study institute, Hotel Thayer, West Point, New York, December 9-12, 1970.* New York: Teachers College Press, 1970.

Watkins, A. V. (Ed). *Syllabus for generic core classes.* Los Angeles: Department of Special Education, California State University, Los Angeles, 1976.

Whitecroft, C. J. Motoric engramming for sensory deprivation or disability. *Exceptional Children,* 1972, *38,* 475-478.

Wyatt, K. E. One Dickens of a Christmas Carol. In F. P. Connor, J. R. Wald, and M. J. Cohen (Eds.), *Professional preparation for educators of crippled children; proceedings of a special study institute, Hotel Thayer, West Point, New York, December 9-12, 1970.* New York: Teachers College Press, 1970.

6 Educational programs

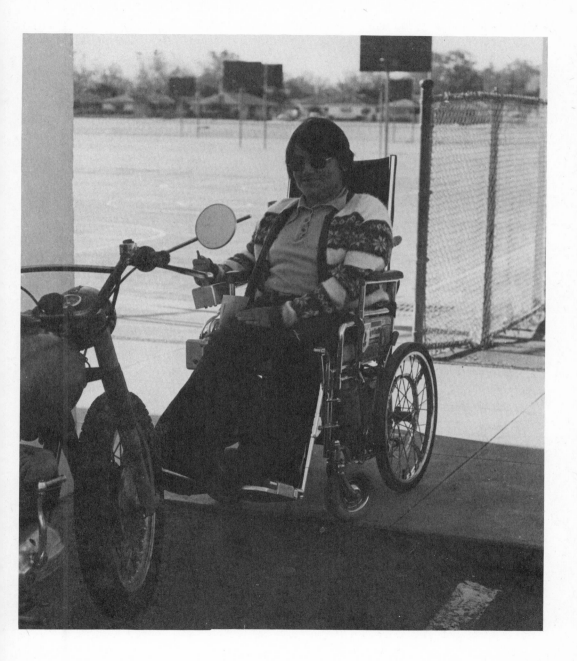

HISTORICAL PERSPECTIVE

In the beginning, *there was nothing.* In this one statement it is possible to find the majority of the history of organized education for children with physical disabilities. The primary goal for most individuals with physical disabilities in our history has been one of survival. Education is a meaningful experience only if one is present to participate in it and there is some expectancy for its use. High mortality, lack of need felt by the general public for the provision of services, a lack of knowledge about the characteristics of those with disabilities, ignorance, unconcern, and out-of-sight, out-of-mind attitudes have all contributed to a historical educational void.

The year 1920 seems to be the turning point for educational services for children with physical disabilities (Cruickshank, 1975; Gearheart and Weishahn, 1976). From this time on, special facilities, including hospital schools, treatment centers, and special education schools and classes, have come into existence on a widespread basis. The evolution has been slow, with a rather short history (not quite 60 years), and is continuing today in light of ever-renewing evaluations of educational systems and the services they provide. Two major factors seem to have contributed to this growth and development of special education services: (1) America's massive involvement in world wars and other armed international conflicts and (2) the organization of parents for the rights of their children.

The nonmilitary and nonpolitical results of America's war involvements during this time helped to bring about a more positive consciousness and awareness of the existence of physical disability. The war efforts created thousands of persons with disabilities who, by the very fact of their survival, had to be confronted by the peoples for which such physical loss was acquired. An exact cause-effect relationship between confrontation with the war-disabled person, and society's recognition of the need to deal with physical disability will probably never be established to the point of satisfactory generalization. However, the large numbers of veterans with disabilities who returned to society, their need to find a place in society, and a need for society to accept the veteran with a disability all had an impact on the awareness and recognition of what disabilities were and what would need to be provided for the disabled person's re-entry into the social and vocational milieu.

At about this same time, parents of children with disabilities were beginning to organize into groups. These organizations were beginning to demand and lobby for services, including educational provisions, that had been denied to them and their children for so long. Their demands carried the force of conviction and later, the force of law. Through their direct efforts it became known that their special children needed not only education, but special education to meet the needs that were obviously not being met in the regular public school environment. This jolting of sensibilities began a period of special education, teacher training, research and development, judicial and legislative decisions, and financial commitment unprecedented in history.

SPECIAL EDUCATION PLACEMENT

Models that have been proposed for the delivery of educational services to children with exceptional needs have been based on the degree of disability and on the educational requirements needed to meet the needs (Deno, 1970). These models, which have been used as generalized schemes for service delivery and administration, are continuums of placement; at the *highest* end of the continuum the child with exceptionality would be placed in a regular education setting, and at the *lowest end* of the continuum service would be provided for the child who was homebound. Placement along the continuum would depend on the disability of the child and his/her needs for care. Although such continuums serve as a paradigm for consideration on a hypothetical level, they often do not reflect the true picture of actual services. Based on incidence figures, there are more children with exceptionalities who are not being served through special education than there are those who are being served. And, for the population of school-aged children with physical disabilities, there are fluctuations in school attendance by grade level and type of setting (Best, 1977; Cruickshank, 1975).

Rather than look at a hierarchical structure for service delivery, then, the following discussion focuses on settings strictly within the realm of special education. Considerations of educational placement for children with disabilities in regular education classes or schools is discussed later in this chapter. The placement services discussed here are probably the least desirable for interaction and integration with normal able-bodied peers, but this description of placement is probably more realistic than other models in that it may be more reflective of where the majority of children with physical disabilities are being served. It is here hypothesized that the following list is representative of where children are placed in descending order of absolute population numbers:

Special schools
Special classes
Homebound programs
Hospital or residential facilities

Special schools

Infant and preschool programs. Not often associated with a public school system, the centers or "schools" for infants and preschool-aged children with physical disabilities may be part of the services offered by organizations such as the United Cerebral Palsy Association; they may be found within hospitals or universities; or they may be private schools developed by parents of children with disabilities. These infant and preschool programs include children who have identified physical disabilities and children who for a variety of physical or medical, or social or economic reasons may be considered to be "at risk" and in need of intervention. Most of these programs also involve one or both of the parents as a part of the terms of enrollment of the child. Stimulation of motor abilities, perceptual and perceptual-motor activities, socialization, and language development are part of an intensive effort to provide the child with an opportunity to grow and develop to the fullest extent within his/her capabilities.

This early intervention helps on two fronts: (1) it is purposeful preparation for later learning experiences, including activities associated with school learning, and (2) it requires involvement of the parent. This latter feature of the infant and preschool programs is significant because of the opportunities it provides for parents (and particularly the mother as the primary care-giver) to be a part of the learning process of the child. This involvement may be especially welcomed in the face of feelings of desperation, fear, guilt, and loneliness experienced by the parents of the child with a physical disability. Parents have the opportunity in these settings to meet as a group with one another and with staff to learn about their child, his/her problems, and methods of handling the child at home. In many cases, this group serves as a forum for sharing concerns and ideas for successful family functioning. It is no small matter for a family to learn to adjust to the needs of the child with a physical disability and to maintain or regain a social-emotional equilibrium.

Elementary schools. What distinguishes a special school from all others is often evident from the street: the name of the school (for example, "The J. J. Smith School for Crippled Children"). This official advertisement of differences is hardly necessary and yet is often encountered. Why not just plain "P. S. 98" or "Smith School"?

Special schools for children with physical disabilities are characterized by a variety of special features:

Barrier-free architecture
Specially trained staff and faculty
Medical treatment facilities
Special equipment and materials
Special transportation
Curriculum and program modifications

To discuss each of these features in a special school is extremely difficult because of the number of variations existing from school to school, district to district, and region to region. Rather than a catalog of all the features of a special school, a description of the day in the life of an elementary school–aged child is presented. This description is intended to be illustrative only, but it is well within the range of possibilities for any given school or child. John, the child described here, has cerebral palsy of the athetotic type. He has quadriplegic involvement and uses a wheelchair most of the time. He can walk but with great difficulty, and he confines his walking to his home at this time. John is in the fifth grade and functions at this grade level in some of his academic subjects. The following is John's school day:

Time	Activity
6:00 AM	John gets up earlier than most children because of the extra time required for him to take care of his dressing, toileting and washing, and eating. Besides, the bus comes by the house to pick him up at 7:30; if he's late, it leaves without him and his mother has to take him to school on her way to work. This puts an extra burden on her, and John knows it. She usually doesn't say too much about it, though, except when everyone has slept in and the house is in the uproar of mad dashing about because everything is running late. Today, however, everything seems to be going rather smoothly, and John is ready for the bus with 5 minutes to spare.
7:46 AM	The bus is late! John's mother was getting a bit worried because she can't leave for work until John is off to school; and the later it gets, the worse the traffic is. John notices that the bus is not the one he usually takes and is told by the driver, Mr. Wallace, that "old 164" had a break in the hydraulic system that operates the lift for the wheelchairs. This doesn't particularly concern John except that he notices that this bus doesn't have a lift, and the side-opening doors don't look wide enough to accommodate his wheelchair. Mr. Wallace seems to notice this, too, but John's only clue to the difficulty the bus driver has is the unusual grunting of the driver as he pulls and lifts John up into the bus. After the chair is braked and fastened into position so that it won't roll when the bus is moving, John notices that Mr. Wallace is sweating a lot. As John looks at his watch, he is aware that there are four more stops; getting to school on time is doubtful today.
8:50 AM	Not too bad! The bus is scheduled to arrive at 8:45, which usually gives John enough time to be unloaded and to get the flag from the office for the morning flag-raising ceremony. Not today; the flag is already up and not upside down, like it was the last time he was late. However, because the bus was late, it is the last in line of the six buses at the loading ramp; this means that John has to wheel himself the full length of the ramp in order to meet his teacher, Mrs. Raeburn, and his classmates at their appointed place at the front of the school. As he wheels past the kindergarten and first grade kids, John notices that some of them look tired, and he remembers when he was younger and would be tired when he got to school. It just takes a lot out of you to get up so early and ride the bus for so long. John was always grateful that his first grade teacher let his class have a sort of rest time or quiet period before they really began their work. It doesn't seem so bad now, though.

8:58 AM   Mrs. Raeburn and the class head down the hall toward their room, which is at the far end of the building. Ordinarily, this doesn't make a whole lot of difference, but the long ramp trip and the fact that he has to go to PT and OT today result in more trips up and down the halls than he would really like to make. John really likes Mrs. Raeburn; she is younger than his mother and just recently married a man she met at the university while taking a night class. She says the class has something to do with teaching, and she sometimes tries out new arithmetic stuff on the class.

9:10 AM   John's class begins after lunch money has been taken and the attendance cards have been sent down to the office by one of the sixth grade kids. The first thing each morning, John and the rest of the class begin their reading work. All of the kids in the class have a folder on their desk put there by Mrs. Raeburn with a list of activities for the day. Mrs. Raeburn develops these lists with each kid on Friday for the week to follow. She calls them contracts, but John sees them simply as lists of things to do. This is OK, though, because it helps John know what it is he needs to do each day. During reading, it is sometimes hard for John to concentrate because of the two kids in the class who do their work with special electric typewriters. They have to use them because they can't write well enough for anyone to read their work. The typewriters have special plates over the keys so that it's hard to hit more than one letter at a time. John used the typewriter once and thought it was fun and was just a little sorry that his own handwriting could be read. Reading has not been a difficult subject for John to handle, and he doesn't know why, except that it is something he and his family have always done at home. (Arithmetic is another matter!) During reading, three of John's classmates leave the room to work with a special teacher in Room 22. She's there to help kids with special problems. Two of John's other friends in the class are in therapy, and one is seeing the speech teacher during the first part of the morning. It sometimes makes Mrs. Raeburn a little angry that so many of the kids are coming and going so much, especially during reading, but she says that scheduling is a problem no matter what time of day it is and that things like therapy and speech are just as important as reading. John is glad that he doesn't go to therapy until the afternoon, because he likes working on reading and arithmetic in the mornings, when there aren't so many kids in the class. John notices today that, with two of the kids absent, two in therapy, one with the speech teacher, and three with the special teacher in Room 22, there are only seven others in the room. This is just fine with him, since it gives him more time to ask Mrs. Raeburn or Mrs. Crane, the aide, questions about his assignments.

10:00 AM   John has to go to the bathroom. This is not something that he likes to do at school, because it's sometimes hard for him to move from his wheelchair to the toilet, adjust his clothes, do what he has to do, and reverse the process. He hates to have Mrs. Crane help him, because he is beginning to be pretty uncomfortable about having a woman help him with going to the bathroom. It is even getting embarrassing having his mother help him, although she has been helping him as long as he can remember. He would really like to be able to wait until recess to go, when Mr. Walters could help him. John wishes that the school had more male aides, but Mr. Walters is the only one in the school; and he's often busy helping the teacher and kids in his own class. The extra-wide stall in the bathroom isn't occupied when he gets there, so there is plenty of room for the wheelchair. John can use the grab bars next to the toilet to help himself out of the wheelchair. He's really glad these bars are there, because it makes the problem of transfer a bit easier for him. His folks put them in the bathroom at home 3 years ago, and this has helped a lot, especially since he no longer knocks over the pretty soap dishes that his mother keeps on the sink, which he would sometimes grab for support. Fortunately, John experiences very little difficulty in toileting today and is soon ready to return to the classroom.

10:15 AM   The 15 minutes that it took John to go to the bathroom were a part of the school day he likes the most: current events. Mrs. Raeburn makes sure everyone has an opportunity to contribute, even the kids who have bad speech problems. This activity comes just before recess and is a great break in the morning work. Mrs. Raeburn has made John and his classmates feel that what they say is important, so everyone in the class likes this part of the morning. Sometimes they talk about things other than news stories: things like baseball, movies, television, or music.

10:30 AM   Recess! For John and most of the other kids in the school, this is the first real opportunity they have during the day to socialize and play. Many of the kids in John's class can play a modified type of softball; some play table games; others play four-square; and others just get together in groups and visit. John would like to play ball, but he can't wheel his chair fast enough around the bases, and his batting isn't that good, so he pretty much sits on the sidelines and makes comments, sometimes quite loudly, about the feats of his classmates. John has learned not to be too adventuresome on the climbing equipment on the playground. A year ago, he managed to get himself out of his wheelchair and start climbing up the monkey bars. He lost his grip and fell through the bars like a ball traveling through a pinball machine and landed on the rubber-cushioned pad underneath the bars with quite a bang. Although not hurt too badly—a few big bruises—he told himself that he wouldn't try *that* again. Some of the kids on the playground are restricted from climbing on the bars and from playing contact games such as baseball because of their disabilities; John has not had such restrictions placed on him by his doctor but his attempt and failure were enough to last a long time.

10:50 AM   After recess Mrs. Raeburn has planned for everyone to do arithmetic. This is John's most difficult subject, and he frequently has trouble with some of the things that Mrs. Raeburn is talking about. John sometimes visits with the special teacher in Room 22 during arithmetic time. She seems to have a special way of explaining things and of helping him that makes him feel good about what he is doing. This year has been somewhat more difficult for John, though, because just when he thought he was doing all right, the school system, or somebody, decided that everyone had to learn about the metric system; and this has set him back a few notches. He doesn't care whether he learns about centimeters or not. Mrs. Raeburn has gotten a lot of materials from the district resource center that John can measure with and compare sizes and lengths, and things like that, but it doesn't seem to do much good. Maybe that's why Mrs. Raeburn is going to night classes at the university—so that she can help John and his classmates learn the new system.

11:50 AM   The past hour has passed rather uneventfully. All of the kids in John's class have worked on arithmetic, and no one has been out of the room for therapy or anything else. Now, everyone is helping put materials away for the art class, which will begin after lunch and the noontime recess.

NOON   John eats lunch in the school cafeteria with some of his friends who have brought their lunch from home. Some of the kids in the lower grade classes are eating with the assistance of the aides, and one of the younger kids is being helped by one of the school's occupational therapists. John knows of no one in his fifth grade class who needs help eating, but he has a friend in a combination fifth-sixth grade class who still has difficulty with some foods and needs the aide from his room to help him. John has often thought about how hard some of the aides in his school work. Some of them work with groups of kids in class, on lessons such as reading or arithmetic, and also have to find time to help with toileting and eating. After lunch, John and his friends go to the playground area for the noontime recess. Because it is hotter now than it was in the morning, he decides to stay in the shade of the building and talk with some of his friends. It is difficult to visit with his friends when they are not at school, because they live so far away from one another. Although John may use the phone at home to call his friends, his folks don't like the monopoly that he sometimes seems to create with the use of the phone. And, besides, talking on the phone isn't quite the same as visiting in person.

12:50 PM   The PT room is down two rather long halls at the opposite end of the school from where John's classroom is located. By leaving the playground a little before the bell rings, John figures he should be able to get to therapy at just about the right time for his 1:00 o'clock session. PT couldn't come at a worse time as far as he's concerned. Right after lunch for the next 3 days, his class and the combination fifth-sixth grade class are painting the backdrops for the spring school play. His teacher and the teacher of the other class have found a way for all the kids in both classes to participate in the scenery painting, and this has been a lot of fun—certainly a lot more fun than his PT exercises will be. John wheels around the treatment mats, toward the parallel bars, which he will use to help in his walking practice. Even though walking is difficult for him, the therapist says John should practice it more, because she thinks that he will someday be taken out of the wheelchair by the clinic doctor. This will please his folks, but John will miss the wheelchair; to be honest, he is just a bit lazy.

1:30 PM   The two classes are just starting to clean up the art materials when John returns to the room from PT. John won't have therapy tomorrow, and he is looking forward to participating in the painting again. When he enters the room, Mrs. Raeburn asks him if this isn't the afternoon that he also has OT. John replies in the affirmative, wishing he didn't have to make the long trip back down the two halls at 2:00 o'clock, not only because he's getting tired, but also because of the spring play practice. Mrs. Raeburn says she will call the OT office and see if John can reschedule his treatment session for another time that won't interfere with the play practice. John's relief can almost be heard when he learns that OT will gladly switch treatment times. During the class practice of the spring play, a group of visitors from some organization comes by to visit the room. Usually this type of interruption doesn't bother John, but he is somewhat more conscious of the visitors today because of the play rehearsal. He used to be bothered by groups coming to look at his school and class all the time. It seemed as though he were in a goldfish bowl and people were coming to stare at him. John has gotten used to these visits for the most part, but he wishes this group would go away fast because he's nervous enough about saying his lines correctly without having a bunch of people just stare at him. He hopes it will be different during the play. Then, people will come to see him and his friends as characters in a play. Mrs. Raeburn says that being nervous about being on the stage is natural.

2:30 PM John and his classmates have gathered all of their books, coats, and other personal belongings together to take with them to the auditorium, where they are going to meet with the adaptive PE teacher. By taking all of their personal stuff with them, they won't have to go back to the room after working with the adaptive PE teacher before getting on the bus. The adaptive PE teacher is helping the class with a dance they will be doing as part of the spring play. Although the dance seems kind of dumb to John, he goes along with the rest of the kids because he knows it is an important part of the play.

3:00 PM The class practices the dance right up to the last bell of the day. John and his friends leave the auditorium for the loading ramp, and he's thankful that he doesn't have to travel a long way to get on the bus. His bus is the first one in line this afternoon, and he notices that it's the regular one. The hydraulic lift is working fine now, and John is sure that Mr. Wallace is glad about that.

4:00 PM The trip home is quiet this afternoon, and John is thankful for that. He feels that he has had a long day and would just as soon not be bothered with a lot of shouting and talking on the way home. The other thing for which John is thankful today is that Mrs. Raeburn has not given any homework to do tonight. His mother is home when he gets there, and all he wants to do is go to his room and rest a bit before getting involved in family activities. His grandmother is coming to the house tonight to stay with him, because tonight is parent guild meeting night; and his folks like to attend whenever they can. That's great as far as John is concerned, because his grandmother will let him watch whatever he wants to on television.

High schools. Special high schools that stand as separate units from other schools appear to be relatively few in number. Where they do exist, these schools are not unlike high schools for abled-bodied students. Classrooms are not much different from what would be expected in any other high school. There are likely to be wood shops, metal shops, home economics departments with fully equipped kitchens, gymnasiums where a full, though modified, program of physical education activities are scheduled, and the traditional locker areas that seem to be the meeting place for all students everywhere. The business education department may be equipped with various typewriters as well as other business machines. Science labs are not uncommon. Physical therapy and occupational therapy may or may not have separate treatment facilities on the grounds of the special high school. The presence of these treatment facilities may depend on the availability of treatment centers elsewhere in the community. At this point in the student's life, therapy may not be as frequent or as intense as at the elementary school level; hence, outpatient therapy services may be all that is necessary.

The special high school may include some of the special characteristics of the special elementary school. These would include architectural and building features such as extra-wide hallways and doors; an abundance of handrails, both in the classrooms and in the bathrooms; and lowered water fountains, telephones, and bathroom fixtures. Special instructional equipment—electric typewriters, with and without guide plates over the keys; automatic electric page turners; and other appliances that might facilitate learning—may also be seen in these schools. The schools are likewise equipped with loading ramps to receive the special buses that are used to transport some of the students to school. However, there is another feature of the special high school that is not unlike that of high schools for able-bodied students: the parking lot. Many students with disabilities may have cars with special adaptive driving equipment, or students may have acquired driving skills without special equipment, so that the parking lot is likely to be filled with that great American sign of teenage independence: the car.

The most notable feature of the special high school is the lack of characteristics distinguishing it from a regular-type high school. The school academic program is not that much different from a regular high school in that it offers a college preparatory curriculum, a vocational curriculum, and a curriculum for those with learning problems or for those who are slow learners. Student government, class plays, dances, proms, and carnivals are a part of the high school program, as are competitive sports, pep rallies, and cheerleaders.

If all of this is the same, then why are there special high schools? Or, what *does* make the difference? These special high schools, as noted earlier, are few in number and exist primarily in large urban areas where there is a significantly large population of students with disabilities to warrant such a school and/or where students have disabilities to such a degree that they are unable to participate in a regular school program, or to a degree that attendance in such programs is physically impractical. The question of "Why are there special high schools?" may be looked at, if not adequately answered, from several points of view: (1) the school exists, and there is a commitment to this type of special education services and philosophical management of disability; (2) the students are physically disabled and/or educationally retarded to the extent that participation in a regular school setting would be unreasonable or a detriment to their own growth, education, and welfare; and (3) special services are available for independent life training, including work-training programs and personal living skills.

•   •   •

Regarding the presence of special schools in the community, several points should be kept in mind. There are some students who need the special programs and services offered by these schools. On the other hand, special schools should not become a haven or dumping ground for students who can, and should, be placed in regular school settings. When this occurs, special schools tend to foster the protective atmosphere so often imposed on persons with physical disabilities. The sheltered surroundings of the special school is not conducive to the learning that comes from interaction with the able-bodied population. It will be difficult for students to leave the protection of the special schools and take their own places in society if there have not been sufficient opportunities to participate in that society in a meaningful way during the school years. A special school education may indeed tend to avoid the blows from the school of hard knocks that will follow the termination of this education.

Special classes

Special classes for students with physical disabilities are little more than a variation on the theme of the special school. What distinguishes this type of placement from the special school—and what sets it apart—is the location of the special class: on the grounds (and often in the same building) of a regular school facility. For both elementary and secondary school–aged students, this placement practice puts the child with a disability in an environment with normal, able-bodied peers. The special class may be one of two kinds: a self-contained room or a resource-homeroom.

In the self-contained room placement, students with disabilities receive all of their academic activities in the special class. There may be interaction with able-bodied peers during nonacademic activities, such as lunch breaks, recesses, or other special activities involving total school participation. The self-contained room concept does little for the goal of integrating students so that they can learn to work and live together with their unique qualities. This type of special class may run the risk of stigmatization of the students to the degree that they are made even more special in the eyes of their schoolmates. This is particularly possible if the "special kids" receive extra services not available to the entire school population. Special consideration such as field trips, materials, and other preferential treatment by the school may be viewed by other students as unfair or condescending.

The special class in a regular school setting that serves as a resource-homeroom is one of the best methods of providing a regular education environment to students with special needs and still provide the special services made necessary by their disabilities. These classes openly establish contact with students and teachers in the other rooms and classes in the school. In the resource-homeroom, students participate in regular education classes for part of their school day and in the special class for one or more periods of the day. The special class in this arrangement may be used as a center for special help or materials or as a homeroom for counseling, advisement, or other special needs.

Before special class placement for the integration of students for part or the majority of the school day is implemented, certain prerequisites should be considered. The student should be physically capable of caring for his/her needs, including the ability to be mobile within the setting. This mobility criterion should not exclude the use of a wheelchair or crutches. The building in which the special class is housed should be modified to reduce or eliminate architectural barriers for ease of travel by the student with special mobility needs. If the student is in need of therapy, arrangements may need to be made for outpatient treatment or for released time during the school day for treatment off-campus. The possibility of bringing treatment to the school by an itinerant therapist may also be explored. Perhaps one of the most crucial aspects of this integration school plan concerns cooperation including the school administrators. The special class teacher who has students participating in classes other than his/her own will need to be available to colleagues for consultation, encouragement, and support. This support should not only be in form of attending to problems that arise, but should also be in the nature of providing suggestions that may be helpful to colleagues in developing in-service education and that may help in the establishment of goodwill for the children. Maintaining a distance from the teachers to which the special class students are sent may result in a feeling of abandonment by the regular education teacher. A cooperative arrangement by the special class teacher to accept some of the able-bodied students in his/her class for a variety of lessons or activities may help the staff establish a feeling of mutual contribution and success for one another's students and the total school program.

Homebound programs

Programs for students who are homebound fall into two main categories: instruction by the home teacher and telephone instruction. In either type of program, students are unable to attend school for a variety of reasons. Students who may receive home instruction are those who

> . . . are so severely handicapped as to be unable to profitably attend either a regular school or a special class; are confined to their homes . . . for a limited period, following a traumatic episode or surgical procedure; suffer from a chronic disabling illness; have a medical condition which makes transportation unfeasible; being handicapped, find no suitable school program available to them in their district. (Sehler, 1973. pp. 5-6)

Pregnant school-aged girls may also receive home instruction (Outland and Gore, 1969), although many districts provide for instruction of these girls in special classes or maternity homes (Howard, 1975). These special classes provide the expectant mother with ongoing medical care, a continuation of education, and counseling services. Still, according to Howard,

> The choice of whether to remain in regular school, attend adult school, enroll in special classes for young mothers, or receive home tutoring should be the

student's. It should be based on a genuine assessment of each individual's situation, not some arbitrary classification of where or how pregnant girls or young parents should be educated. (p. 89)

For all students who are homebound, medical evaluation should be the prime criteria for this placement; and the students should receive instruction in this manner only as long as it is medically necessary. Reevaluation of the students physical condition should be done regularly, so that exclusion from school attendance is at a minimum.

Instruction by the home teacher. The role of the home teacher is not unlike that of any other teacher. The teacher who provides instruction in the home has additional responsibilities however, that are not often encountered by either regular education teachers or other special education teachers. The home teacher must be responsive to (1) the educational needs of each of his/her students, (2) the ongoing educational program of the school from which the student was previously enrolled, (3) the actual teaching for which the teacher is directly responsible, and (4) the psychosocial needs of the student and the parent who is contact with the teacher during each visit. This multitude of responsibilities requires the teacher to be in contact with the student's previous teacher in order to (1) ensure a continuation of the program of the student; (2) have an awareness of the physical limitations of the child, including the child's strength and tolerance for periods of work; and (3) be knowledgeable about the availability of special materials, curricula, and services that may be necessary or of benefit to each student. The teacher's car becomes a traveling school, resource center, library, and consulting center.

Although the home teacher is able to provide a continuation of the student's educational program within the limits of the student's disability, there are other considerations that may be of more importance such as the social isolation of the student from his/her peers. In a study of the attitudes of homebound high school students toward their return to school, Rusalem and Jenkins (1961) found that the students were more concerned about the social limitations of home instruction than about their educational proficiency. This social isolation may in part, be relieved by the use of telephone instruction for students who are homebound.

Telephone instruction. Telephone instruction, an important trend in home instruction (Best, 1967), provides for the instruction of students in their homes at increased levels of interaction with the teacher and makes available the companionship of others through the equivalent of telephone conference calls. Through special equipment involving automatic card dialers connected to a console operated by the teacher (Fig. 6-1), students may "attend" school on a daily basis and participate in group discussions and lessons or in individual conferences with the teacher as needed. The teacher can put some class members " on hold" to give individual or small-group help or lessons to others as required by the needs of the students and the grade level of their program. The lightweight headset required for each student does not interfere with the use of the home telephone and allows the student the free use of both hands in the pursuit of daily lessons. Not unlike

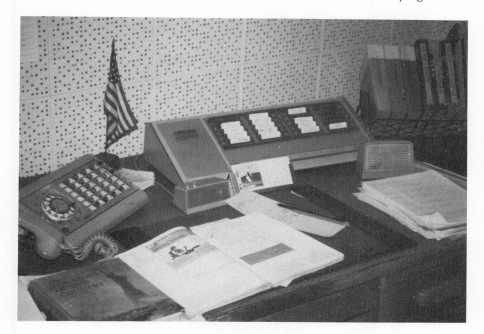

Fig. 6-1. Automatic card dialer.

attendance in any elementary or high school program, the student—depending on the grade level—may receive all of his/her instruction from one teacher, as would be the case in a self-contained elementary school class, or the student may be on a departmentalized telephone teaching arrangement, which would be analogous to the several subjects or academic departments found in a high school curriculum. In this latter arrangement, several telephone teachers would be responsible for the establishment and arrangement of schedules so that each student on the telephone instruction network would be assigned to a particular teacher at a given time for freshman English, second-year algebra, or whatever subject and level would be appropriate.

Residential and hospital programs

Residential and hospital programs are grouped together here, not because of any particular similarity in their programs, but because of the relatively low numbers of students found in each of these programs in comparison with the programs previously mentioned. Each of these programs and the facilities in which they are housed are unique and represent a different level of care and educational program.

Residential facilities. Residential facilities, which may be a part of a state residential and care hospital or school system, or part of the service provided by a private agency, offer a variety of services and functions: education, social interaction and companionship, work training, counseling, medical treatment, educational and psychological diagnoses, and residence for board and physical care. Whether a part of a state system, or a function of a private agency, the principle drawback of such a care facility is its isolation from the world within which it exists. In spite of this drawback, however, the residential facility may be of benefit to the child and the family for a variety of reasons.

When the child has a disability to such a severe degree that he/she is unable to participate and benefit from a public school program, the residential care facility may be an alternative placement. When this same child may not be capable of receiving the support of the family because of the physical or emotional drain caused by the child's presence, placement in a residential care facility may be opted for. When the child with a disability lives in a region such as a rural area or sparsely populated state that does not have special education facilities to meet the child's educational or physical treatment needs, a state or regional school may provide for the child.

In those instances wherein an individual who is severely disabled is placed in a residential facility, the educational program will be commensurate with his/her physical and mental abilities. This may mean a preacademic, academic, or self-care curriculum depending on individual assessment and goal direction. For the student who is at a severe level of physical and mental involvement, the curriculum may not be significantly different from that found in a special class or school.

A final word about this type of facility: Although such facilities serve a purpose in the treatment, education, and care of persons with disabilities, the absence of family and friends and the home environment may have a serious impact on the psychological well-being of the individual. The fears and anxieties caused by separation and loss of family togetherness and support may be such that adjustment to this placement arrangement will be unsatisfactory. Family and friends, as well as staff at the facility, must make every effort to provide the resident with the support necessary to alleviate feelings of abandonment and to encourage a sense of worthiness and self-respect in the individual despite his/her place of residence.

Hospital instruction. The hospital teacher faces one of the greatest challenges in the teaching profession. Without too much difficulty, one could get caught up in the mechanics of teaching in a situation where medical treatment is the prime reason for placement. The hospital teacher must be able to provide an educational environment and learning experience in a children's ward, in a room or rooms set aside by the hospital as the "school," or at the bedside of the student-patient who, because of prosthetic and/or life support equipment, is unable to move to a more traditional classroom setting. Furthermore, the teacher must be responsive to the treatment, surgical, and/or recuperative needs of the student-patient and be able to make adjustments in the daily schedule for rest periods, radiographic studies, laboratory visits, and a myriad of other interruptions. These medically oriented activities are then put into the perspective of the student-patient's educational needs and level of performance and the teacher's need to maintain, and provide an opportunity for, academic progress. These medical-educational functions challenge the teacher in meeting the purposes of hospital instruction as enumerated by Sehler (1973):

1. Compensate for loss of in-school experience—with special emphasis on academic and social development.
2. Adjust instructional efforts to a student's individual needs, abilities and interests, on the basis of appropriate performance objectives.
3. Evaluate educational status, and interpret the progress of each pupil enrolled.
4. Provide a continuum of services which prepares the child to resume school attendance as smoothly as circumstances permit.
5. Investigate and/or initiate avenues of rehabilitation open to each student.
6. Provide a supportive and interpretive liaison service among parents, school personnel, and student.
7. Coordinate and provide counseling regarding use of the services of public and private community agencies and other resources.
8. Provide continuity to the mental, social, emotional and physical development of . . . [the hospitalized] child. (p. 1-2)

In addition to the purposes listed above, there is yet another aspect of interaction that must be given equal, if not greater consideration in regard to the welfare of the child: the child's feelings about hospitalization. In the case of admittance into an acute hospital setting, the child may be experiencing pain, serious illness, or trauma from accidental injury. In addition, the child may be unaccustomed to the sights, sounds, smells, people, and other strange and frightening things that surround and invade the child's privacy as a person. Strange food served in a different way, strange people doing strange things to him/her and a strange-looking bed— the child is confronted by all these and builds up anxieties and fears that may be compounded when the child realizes that mother and father have to go home and he/she is to be left alone in this place. Separation and abandonment become real and make adjustment to illness, recuperation, and finally school-type activities even more difficult.

The child who is admitted to a chronic care hospital for ongoing treatment or recurring illness may have different feelings about hospitalization from the child who is admitted for the first time to an acute care setting. However, these feelings may be no less intense and require attention for conflict resolution. Dealing with feelings of loneliness, boredom, and uncertainty about the future may be more important than attending to educational concerns.

School and play are an integral part of the lives of children. And because this integration of school and play is so important, it may serve to reduce the anxieties of children and help pave the way toward treatment success and reintegration into the familiar life from which the child has come. "A medical facility should provide more than just medical treatment. It should look to the well-being of the whole person, whether a patient or a parent or a child of a patient" (Azarnoff and Flegal, 1975, p. 10).

MAINSTREAMING PRACTICES

The first consideration that should be mentioned about the concept of mainstreaming is that *it is not new*. The decade following Dunn's (1968) article questioning special education placement of mildly handicapped children has been one of evaluating, reevaluating, and energizing the movement of children with a variety of disabilities into or back into the regular classroom. The movement has been popularized, and the catch phrase "the *mainstream* of education" has been employed to describe the educational placement of children with disabilities in classes with their normal peers. Some form of integration has occurred for probably as long as 30 years, and Force (1956) studied the effects of the integration of children with physical disabilities in classes with their normal peers almost 25 years ago. What does seem to be new about this current movement is the widespread support it has received both inside and outside the field of special education. This support has been formalized by recent legislation. The effects of PL 94-142, the Education for All Handicapped Children Act, has been such that the integration of children with disabilities in classes with normal peers will not now happen in a hit-or-miss manner; it is now "the law of the land."

Mainstreaming, the educational process whereby the child with a disability receives part or all of his/her education with normal peers, will not eliminate the need for special classes and special schools. There are some children with disabilities who are so severely impaired and/or have such a multiplicity of disabilities that their special education needs cannot be met in the regular class. For children who are able to participate in this process, however, and this includes children at all grade levels and throughout the range of disability types (Best, 1977), the opportunity to interact and share meaningful life experiences, including the give and take of everyday social participation, with normal peers will benefit all involved. What may happen is that the fears and uncertainties from a lack of previous socialization will be broken down or become nonexistent. On the other hand, what may also occur is outright confrontation of prejudice and the need to combat it not only for the development of tolerance, but also for the acceptance and mutual respect for the qualities and abilities of both the able-bodied and the disabled participants.

For mainstreaming to be a success, and there is no guarantee that it will be, there needs to be an opportunity for those who will be involved to learn about the process. The student's both able-bodied and disabled, their parents, and the teachers and administrators in both regular and special education will need to establish a communication network that will foster the mainstreaming process. This can be accomplished with minimum difficulty through education and training at the pre-service and in-service levels. The implementation of mainstreaming should signal a professional mandate for all educators to become involved and informed about what strategies will enhance and provide for the greatest measure of success of this placement and learning process.

NONTRADITIONAL EDUCATIONAL PROGRAMS
Open education

With the success of the British informal schools, open education as an alternative form of curricular organization and management and as a means for developing social responsibility in students involved in the program has been welcomed and met with considerable success in the United States. This type of placement is not to be confused with lack of structure or freedom from responsibility.

> Open education is an approach to education that is open to change, to new ideas, to curriculum, to scheduling, to use of space, to honest expressions of feeling between teacher and pupil, and between pupil and pupil, and open to children's participation in significant decision making in the classroom. (Stephens 1974, p. 27)

As an alternative form of educational placement, open education as defined above seems made to order for children with physical disabilities.

Special class and special school placement have all but ignored the open education approach to learning for children with special needs. This has been particularly the case in the educational placement of children with physical disabilities. As with many educational strategies that have gained popularity in the profession, bits and pieces of open education have been tried with varying degrees of success and failure. What often occurs is the initiation of the plan without the teacher's thorough understanding of it or without the necessary skills or trust established by both the teacher and the students. Since special schools and classes offer a protective environment in which the majority of decisions about educational and physical treatment is made for them, children with physical disabilities often lack the experience of making decisions and taking responsibility for behavior—two of the keystones of open education.

"What if the child decides he doesn't want to read or go to therapy?" This question is not inconsistent with the fears of educators who have not extended to their students the trust needed for them to make their own decisions. However, open education is not without decision making on the part of the teacher and not without structure in the learning process. Therefore, if the teacher is not comfortable letting students make decisions regarding whether or not they should participate in reading or in therapy, the teacher need not make this decision option available for the students.

> The goal of the teacher in an open classroom is to develop pupils' ability to assume more and more responsibility for decision making. Not that all decisions will eventually be made by pupils. We reiterate that *child responsibility does not mean abdication of teacher responsibility.* Varying patterns of re-

sponsibility for different activities will continue to exist. (Stephens, 1974, p. 45)

It seems logical that if practice by students in adding figures together is considered necessary for them to develop a level of expertise commensurate with the demands of number manipulation in adult life, then practice in decision making should also be given the same level of curricular importance. Are special educators guilty of not expecting or wanting for their students the same goals and development of responsibility regular education teachers, or at least regular education teachers who teach in an open classroom setting, want for their students?

Although open education is not suggested as a panacea for the assumed or real ills of traditional classroom organization and management, it is suggested as an alternative that is viable and possible for implementation. Two sets of questions about open education are presented here for the reader's consideration: (1) What have you got to lose? What do you stand to gain? (2) What have the children got to lose? What do the children stand to gain?

Respite homes

Respite homes may be a part of or apart from the educational services provided by a school district. These homes or apartments provide room and board away from the child's home. Two benefits may be seen as a result of the provision of these services: (1) the parents are given a break—respite—from the ongoing and demanding care of a child with a physical disability, and (2) the child is given not only a break from his/her parents but also the opportunity to learn the requirements of living away from their care and shelter. Depending on the ages of the youngsters involved in the program, children who live in respite homes for periods of a few days to several weeks learn to cooperate with other children in the home and to participate in the maintenance of the home, including food shopping, meal preparation and cleanup, and the thousand and one other skills necessary for running a home.

House parents with a background in or knowledge of physical disabilities and independent living skills provide guidance and a learning environment not readily found in traditional school programs. As both a respite from care for parents and a training facility for children, respite homes have the potential for serving and filling a great need in the special community of children with disabilities and their parents.

SUMMARY

The different educational settings that have characterized special education for children with physical disabilities have been identified and discussed. Until recently, the most prominent among these educational placement types has been the segregated school facility. This type of school has been architecturally designed to accommodate the needs of children with physical limitations and has been able to offer the special services of therapists, specially trained teachers, and other professionals within the confines of the facility.

What these segregated school and class settings have offered in addition to special education services, however, is a sheltered atmosphere wherein interaction with a normal peer group has been discouraged if not specifically avoided. PL. 94-142 has now set into motion conditions that will mandate a change more significant in the education of children with physical disabilities than at any other time in the history of public education. With this advent of integrated public education whereby normal children will have the opportunity to interact with those with physical disabilities, education is moving from a commitment to separate but equal education to one of social involvement more realistically parallel to the whole of social circumstance.

The teacher's own choice of program implementation may be limited by the job opportunities available. However, the choice of caring, humaneness, and humanness in the teaching of children should be no choice at all. These qualities should be present regardless of where one teaches.

REFERENCES

Azarnoff, P., and Flegal, S. *A pediatric play program: developing a therapeutic play program for children in medical settings.* Springfield, Ill. Charles C Thomas, Publisher, 1975.

Best, G. A. State provisions for home instruction. *Exceptional Children,* 1967, *34,* 33-36.

Best, G. A. Mainstreaming characteristics of orthopedically handicapped students in California. *Rehabilitation Literature,* 1977, *38,* 205-209.

Cruickshank, W. M. The development of education for exceptional children. In W. M. Cruickshank and G. O. Johnson (Eds.), *Education of exceptional children and youth* (3rd ed.). Englewood Cliffs, N.J.: Prentice-Hall, Inc., 1975.

Deno, E. Special education as developmental capital. *Exceptional Children,* 1970, *37,* 229-237.

Dunn, L. M. Special education for the mildly retarded: is much of it justifiable? *Exceptional Children,* 1968, *35,* 5-22.

Force, D. G., Jr. Social status of physically handicapped children. *Exceptional Children,* 1956, *23,* 104-107; 132.

Gearheart, B. R., and Weishahn, M. W. *The handicapped child in the regular classroom.* Saint Louis: The C. V. Mosby Co., 1976.

Howard, M. *Only human: teenage pregnancy and parenthood.* New York: The Seabury Press, Inc., 1975.

Outland, W. O., and Gore, B. E. *Home and hospital instruction in California.* Sacramento: Department of Education, State of California, 1969.

Rusalem, H., and Jenkins, S. Attitudes of homebound students toward return to regular classroom attendance. *Exceptional Children,* 1961, *28,* 71-74.

Sehler, A. B. (Ed.). *Tips for the development of programs for the homebound and hospitalized.* Council for Exceptional Children: Division of Physically Handicapped, Homebound and Hospitalized. Lansing, Mich.: The Instructional Materials Development Center, Michigan School for the Blind, 1973.

Stephens, L. S. *The teacher's guide to open education.* New York: Holt, Rinehart & Winston, 1974.

7 Curriculum and instructional modifications

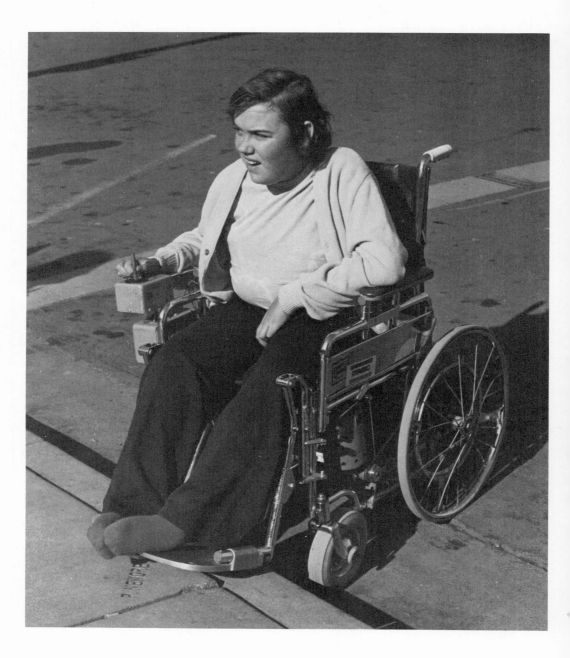

This chapter is not intended as a mini–curriculum guide or a teacher's cookbook on what to do and how to do it. There are however, some suggestions for activities that might be considered by the classroom teacher. The thrust of this book to this point has been, whenever possible, child centered. One of the perspectives of special education should be that each child is indeed special, with unique requirements for learning. Where grouping for activities because of shared levels of performance and/or need is practical, however, these group experiences should be provided.

The special education teacher is blessed by two universal (or almost universal) classroom characteristics: a small class size and a classroom aide. To the envy of regular education teachers, the size of the special class for children with disabilities may be limited because of a variety of factors: the children's age; the types of disability that may be represented in the classroom; or the presence of multiple disabilities, including mental retardation and perceptual or learning disabilities; or a combination of two or more of these factors. This limited population in the classroom enables the teacher to provide for the individualization that is so necessary to the child and his/her learning needs.

The classroom aide may serve to promote and assist the teacher in attaining the maximum of child-centered caring and learning in the classroom. The role of the classroom aide is one that is not always carefully defined or known. Some aides serve little more than as adjunct room custodians, physical care attendants of the children, and "go-fers" (go-fer this and go-fer that: messengers and paper pushers). *What a waste!* Although the just-mentioned activities may be part of the classroom aide's function *as well as that of the teacher's,* the classroom aide is best identified as the teacher's partner in the learning environment of the child. Whether the aide has been trained in a pre-service college program or in a pre-service/in-service school district training program, this person may become a valuable instructional asset to the teacher by providing assistance with individual learning activities and group experiences and by contributing to the ongoing assessment, instruction and psychosocial and physical growth of the children. Care should be taken to nourish and support the mutual professional and personal interactions of the teacher and the aide for the establishment of an educational classroom team.

INFANT AND PRESCHOOL YEARS

The infant and preschool years are the years of discovery: discovery for children as they learn about their bodies and how they function and about their relationship with the world in which they live. This is also a time of discovery for the teacher—to determine the learning levels and growth of the child—and a time of discovery for the parent—to understand what the child is capable of (*and* what the parent is capable of) and can become. It is a period of awakening in everyone. The components of a program for a child with a physical disability are in most ways not unlike those of any early childhood educational experience. What is significantly different about this educational period is the inability of those involved to take for granted the needs of the child and the various experiences that the child may obtain from random sources. For children with disabilities these early educational experiences may prove to be useful in reducing the effects of a disability; or these years may be ones during which direct stimulation will enhance learning potential so that a disability does not result in an unnecessary handicap.

An early educational experience for infants and children with disabilities should include a means of evaluation to determine where the child is developmentally in fine and gross motor abilities, sensory reception and perception, cognitive development, social development, and language development. Although many instruments have been developed that assess and identify levels of functioning in children with disabilities or who may have the potential for impaired learning, there is also some question as to the appropriateness of these instruments as universal guides (Meier, 1976). Therefore, a careful study of the various scales and instruments available should be undertaken before any are recommended for implementation. No child should be bound by the results of an assessment of developmental level. The accuracy of assessment, the actual functioning of the child, and cultural expectations may all interact to provide either a clear picture of functioning or a blurred notion of performance. The teacher who is confronted with the task of providing an educational program for infants and children at these early years is encouraged to find the best possible help and support from a trained team of diagnostic personnel. These professionals, who may include physicians, therapists, psychologists, and teachers, will be able to help determine where the child is and in what direction a program for intervention should be aimed.

The program

At whatever stage an infant or child is found to be functioning, the program should be planned to develop the child's unique potential for growth. The intervention or learning activity should not be hit or miss. A method should be found for providing a sequenced, orderly set of experiences—building experience on top of experience—for the child's growth and development. For example, a child who is functioning at a language level where he/she is capable of little more than saying or signaling yes or no when appropriate should not be expected to respond to questions such as "How did Jane help mother?"

Just as children should not have experiences that are not in a sequential pattern of presentation, neither should they have experiences in isolation. An example of this type of integration of learning activities can be found in language development. Language activities should be a constant; the teacher should speak to the child about the activities that are being experienced. While this language is being expressed, the child might also experience socialization and perceptual discrimination by manipulating different-textured building blocks with the teacher. This interaction of activities is part of a total plan that becomes part of the child's day.

Activities should be planned that provide for socialization of the children in the program, since this may be the first time that the child with a disability has been exposed to children outside of the immediate family. The child should have opportunities to socialize with small groups of children and with adults in the program. It is not unusual to find infants or children with physical disabilities who have limited experiences of socialization with adults other than their parents. Their world has been limited to those few persons who are in the immediate care-giving setting of day-to-day living.

Seeing, hearing, tasting, and touching; putting in and taking out; riding, sitting, standing, walking, running, hopping, falling down and getting up; picking up and putting down; grabbing hold of and releasing; catching and throwing; crying and laughing; and experimenting with the mouth, tongue, and vocal chords all become part of the learning experience. Singing; painting; riding in and on tricycles, wagons, and scooters; water, sand, and block play; dress up and doll play; play involving comparison and conceptualization of sizes, shapes, weights, densities, numbers, and quantities; bead stringing; and toy and game making are also fun activities that aid in learning.

The play environment should include a wide assortment of materials for children to explore and manipulate. Boxes of all shapes and sizes can be played with and in; rugs and other materials of various textures and colors can be used for decorating play areas and play containers and for visual and tactile experiences. Toys that make sounds, move, and have lights are not only fun for children to play with and manipulate, they are also useful for fine and gross motor activity, visual tracking, and visual-motor perceptual skill development.

Resources

There are a wide variety of resources for planning childhood and infant learning experiences and programs. There is no intent to slight any of these resources that may be useful in program development and implementation, but the ones listed below have been found to be of particular interest:

Resource title	Author or organization	Publisher or organization
A Practical Guide to Early Childhood Curriculum	Claudia E. Eliason and Loa T. Jenkins	The C. V. Mosby Co., St. Louis, Mo.
From Birth to One Year	Marilyn M. Segal	The Nova University Play and Learn Program Nova University 3301 College Ave. Ft. Lauderdale, Fla.
From One to Two Years	Marilyn M. Segal and Don Adock	The Nova University Play and Learn Program
Guide to Early Developmental Training	Wabash Center for the Mentally Retarded, Inc.	Allyn & Bacon, Inc., Boston, Mass.
Handling the Young Cerebral Palsied Child at Home	Nancie R. Finnie	E. P. Dutton & Co., Inc. New York, N.Y.

Resource title	Author or organization	Publisher or organization
Infant Stimulation Curriculum	The Developmentally Delayed Infant Education Project	The Nisonger Center for Mental Retardation and Developmental Disabilities, The Ohio State University, Columbus, Ohio
Intervention Strategies for High Risk Infants and Young Children	Theodore D. Tjossem (Ed.)	University Park Press, Baltimore, Md.
Koontz Child Developmental Program Training Activities for the First 48 Months	Charles W. Koontz	Western Psychological Services, Los Angeles, Calif.
Lesson Plans for Enhancing Preschool Developmental Progress	Alton D. Quick and A. Ann Campbell; Project Memphis	Kendall/Hunt Publishing Co., Dubuque, Iowa
Planning Programs for Early Education of the Handicapped	Norman E. Ellis, and Lee Cross (Eds.)	Walker and Co., New York, N.Y.
Teaching Aids and Toys for Handicapped Children	Barbara Dorward	Council for Exceptional Children, Reston, Va.
The Live Oak Curriculum: A Guide to Preschool Planning in the Heterogeneous Classroom	Celeste Myers (Ed.)	Alpha Plus Corp., Circle Preschool 9 Lake Ave. Piedmont, Calif,

Implications for infants or children with multiple disabilities

Infant and preschool educational programs may be a highly significant part of the growth and development of the child with a physical disability and any one or more associated or accompanying disabilities or problems. On entry into a program, several implications of multiple disabilities may be readily evident: motor and sensory development may be severely involved, considerably delayed, or nonexistent; verbal communication may be limited or nonexistent; socialization skills may be limited; personal care functions and abilities may be absent or only partially present—the child may be unable to feed him/herself or may be able to handle only specific kinds of foods; the child may be unable to dress him/herself in whole or in part; and the child may not be toilet trained.

These characteristics of the child with multiple disabilities should not be seen as criteria for program participation; but the child's inability to feed him/herself or to communicate the need to be toileted are part of the child's current level of functioning and become a base for program development for the child by the teacher and the parents. In addition to the learning and socialization activities previously discussed, the limitations of function imposed by multiple disabilities become part of the daily school program.

The child, then, becomes a part of his/her own program. The child, disability, and program become one. This concept serves to provide for the inclusion, rather than the exclusion, of the child from organized learning. Attempts to intervene at an early age of the child may work toward reducing the long-term effects of disability, help promote later success at formalized learning, and eventually lead to higher individualized levels of independence.

Role of the parents

The child cannot be served alone. Parents have one of the largest investments of all. From the beginning, they have needs that are often thwarted or unmet or that must be redefined. For the parents of the infant or child with a physical disability, there must be a period of adjustment to the fact of the presence of disability. This adjustment is made more difficult by the expectations imposed by society for normal child rearing and the implications of these expectations for the child and the family. These expectations require reconciliation of knowledge of the child as a person with knowledge of the disability and its present and possible future implications for the child's functioning. It should not be assumed that this link of the child and the disability will, or even can, be made by the parents. It is not unknown for parents to keep these two entities of child and disability separate in their interactions with the child. The denial of one may or may not be contingent on the denial or acceptance of the other.

Parents may come to the first school setting with a history of fears, guilt, lack of knowledge, anger, and frustration. Many of these feelings may continue to exist and may or may not change in intensity and direction in the years to come. But it is during these early years of school association that parents may come to realize that both they and their child have a future that can be rewarding and fulfilling. As parents want to know more about their child and how they can best develop the child's and their own potential, participation in the school program at both the curricular and extracurricular levels should be encouraged. In many infant and preschool programs, one or both of the parents must be participants in school activities as a condition of the child's enrollment. These activities include assistance in the day-to-day instructional program and membership in parent advisory councils and discussion groups.

> When parents become part of the teaching team, a heartening phenomenon often occurs. The parents experience a new sensitivity and heightened awareness of their own child's individual pattern and rate of growth and development. They sense that learning can and will take place. Moreover, goals and routines devised in the classroom can be taken home for integration into a total family experience. (Wabash Center for the Mentally Retarded, Inc., 1977, p. iv)

Parents of children with special needs should not be considered passive partners in the learning process. It has been through the activities of parents, individually and as groups, that major changes have come about in the services and educational programs in existence today.

ELEMENTARY SCHOOL YEARS

The time period between kindergarten and the sixth grade, and in some instances the eighth grade, is one in which the foundations and major supports of the child's educational attainments will have been built. Traditionally, these are the years during which the basic academic subject areas are taught and learned. It is within this same tradition that the elementary school years of children with physical disabilities should be spent. The curriculum should include reading, arithmetic, language, science, the social studies (history, geography, current events), and those areas that are not thought of as academic, perhaps, but are nevertheless an important part of the curriculum: art, music, and physical education/recreation. Since the subject areas of this proposed curriculum are not unlike those found in any regular educational setting, are there any special concepts regarding the curriculum that are, or should be, different for children with physical disabilities?

In considering the similarity of the curriculum stated as appropriate for normal children and that proposed for special children, one should keep the following in mind: one of the aims of special education for children with physical disabilities is to put itself out of business. That is, special education should strive to provide skills and levels of knowledge for the students within its care that will make them able to participate and compete during their growing years in activities with their able-bodied peers. This will ultimately lead, it is hoped, to the individual's ability to participate as an adult in the activities of the majority society in as independent and satisfying a manner as possible. The ability to develop and use skills in such areas as reading and arithmetic will be needed by children with disabilities for academic survival when they are integrated with their able-bodied peers. For, just as surely as this integration will be accomplished, a student's inability to perform at expected achievement levels will serve to bring about segregation of that student within a physical environment of mutual space sharing. Thus, to ignore "normal" subject areas for children who have the potential and capacity for achievement is to assign them to levels of second-class citizenship. The educational curriculum for children with physical disabilities, whether they are served in a regular or special education setting, should not be the fun-and-games program of a day camp!

Are there special considerations that should be made in the development and implementation of a curriculum for children with disabilities? Yes. Because of the limitations imposed by disability, physical exploration of the environment may be limited, conceptual development may be retarded, intellectual and/or perceptual abilities may not be at age-expected levels, and language may be inappropriate, inarticulate, or inadequately processed. These and other associated problems that combine to form the complex of multiple disabilities do not fit the mold for a standard curriculum or compartmentalization of school-imposed subject matter. For these children, no assumptions can be made about their knowledge level of such concepts as up-down, foreground-background, directionality, symbolization, or quantity. A differential curriculum, then, must be developed based on an assessment of the functioning and capabilities of the child and not on a specific curriculum guideline or set of directions.

The curriculum

The curriculum for children with physical disabilities should include those academic activities and learning experiences that will prove to be the most useful for the individual's eventual growth, development, and independence of functioning. In addition to the content areas of mathematics, reading, language arts, science, and social studies, children with disabilities also need training and specific learning experiences in areas in which they may be deficient because of their disabilities: visual perception, auditory perception, motor and language activities, and socialization and personal interaction skills. The nature of a differential curriculum, then, is based on the level of functioning of a specific child at any given level, grade, or placement in a school setting. Such a curriculum is not *different* for children with physical disabilities so much as it is individually directed. A consideration of the content areas in isolation from one another is one that should be avoided. Within the areas that might be considered of an academic nature there may be, and in all probability should be, elements of perceptual training and experiences in memory development and social and personal exploration.

Mathematics. Throughout the elementary years, children should have the opportunity to experience arithmetical concepts in a sequential manner from the manipulation of concrete objects to the development of abstractions. They should be provided with materials of different sizes, textures, and colors and of varied structures and designs. These materials may be used to develop a sense of quantity, size, type differentiation, directionality, and arithmetical functions and finally may be used to make the leap from manipulation to symbolization and the abstractions of inference and problem solving.

In all phases of mathematical learning, from simple object manipulation to numeral and function notation (the signs for addition, subtraction, and so on) and the everyday activities of measurement as well as money and other quantitative management, the learner should be presented experiences that have meaning and recognizable characteristics within the individual's realm of understanding. As an example, a class store designed to help children learn about counting, money transactions, budgeting, measuring, and so on may have very little meaning for the child with a physical disability (may be wheelchair bound) who, because of the nuisance of his/her physical care, has never been taken to a grocery store or supermarket. Able-bodied infants and children are often taken to the market by a parent for the daily, weekly, or monthly shopping excursion. These children learn about the intricacies of shopping—there are certain sections for meat, certain sections for dairy products, and certain sections for cereal. The exposure of able-bodied children to this type of experience from an early age, seems to be encouraged by the designers of grocery carts who include a place in the cart for the child to sit while the parent does the shopping. When these children go to school and the teacher decides that a class store will help students learn and practice their skills of sorting, money manipulation, and so on, the classroom experience becomes an extension of that of shopping with a parent and tends to reinforce or legitimatize the knowledge gained from trips to the store.

It is not too difficult to imagine the overwhelming nature of a classroom store experience for the child with a disability who has been left at home because of the bother of physical management or because shopping alone may be one of the few respites the parent has from child care. Thus, the teacher must be aware of the possible deprivation of experiences the child with a disability may have and not assume levels of knowledge or activity based on a normal model.

For the child with multiple disabilities, there will in all probability be more factors influencing the learning of mathematical concepts than just the lack of the experience of riding in a grocery cart. Depending on the nature and degree of involvement of the multiple disabilities, the child may have problems in relation to attention, memory, sequence, quantity reversals, sorting, grouping, and communication. In addition, the child may feel frustration at being unable to understand, let alone master, this set of learning experiences, which may have little or no relation to his/her everyday functioning. Patience on the part of the teacher and a striving for lesson appropriateness will be mandatory. No one method of instruction or type of learning is sacred, and certainly no single set of materials will work magic. Within the limits of reason, safety, and appropriateness, if something works, the teacher should use it; if an experience has meaning for the child, the teacher should see to it that it is available.

Reading. There is probably no other subject of formal education that carries as much importance as reading. The ability to master the written or printed symbolization of the language is one of the major priorities of the school. Pressure to succeed is felt by the child and is compounded by the expectations imposed by others and by self-expectations. For both those with and without disabilities, the need for being able to read is obvious. Some children with physical disabilities may have no more of a problem in learning to read than other children. On the other hand, there may be substantial blocks to the acquisition of this skill. The problem often associated with many disabilities may be such that the prerequisites for mastering symbolization of the language are not met. Problems of auditory and visual perception may prevent sound and print discrimination. Deficiencies in memory (for sequence), head and eye control, and attention to task may lead to problems of left-to-right progression, object location, and difficulty in understanding instruction, content, and meaning. These difficulties may occur in various combinations and may be exacerbated by the fact that many children with disabilities lack the experiential background necessary for being able to comprehend what they are reading. In some instances, it is not that the child is unable to understand what a particular word means; rather, because of a lack of experience with the topic, the child does not have a sense of personal recognition or identity (Compton and Bigge, 1977). It is one thing to be able to read about how cold one's feet become from walking in the snow and quite another to associate walking, coldness, and snow as a meaningful experience.

The professional literature is filled with the identification of various methods of teaching reading, assessing reading ability, diagnosing reading problems, and afixing labels to these problems. Whatever the method or technique of choice, it should be remembered that "the principles of teaching reading to children with physically disabling conditions are the same as those for teaching all other children" (Connor, 1975, p. 455). The teacher's skill in teaching reading to children with physical disabilities will need to include the competencies involved in any particular method or group of methods and the ability to make adaptations of materials and techniques for the use of all the children in the class. As an example, for the child whose physical impairment is such that page turning with a hand is impractical, other methods may be experimented with and used: a pointing stick attached to a helmet or hand splint, an electric page turner, or the use of the feet. The child whose speech impairment is so great as to limit verbal communication will need to be provided with a response mode so that both the teacher and the student will be able to communicate process and comprehension. A method used for communication of personal needs by the child with a severe speech impairment can be easily adapted to meet instructional needs so that the child's communication concerning word meaning or story content may be assessed and understood by the teacher. A response system of eye blinks by the child, pointing with the hand or with a head or hand wand, or other forms of gesturing may be utilized both as a means of assessing learning and as a method of furthering the abilities of the child to communicate.

Language arts. Many academic activities are included within the content area of language arts. Spelling, writing, language development, and grammatical structure of the language are often taught as separate subjects or are combined to provide an integrated sense of language learning. In a practical sense, it may be more convenient to combine the areas of reading, language development and structure, and spelling as a total package of language experience. On the other hand, activities such as spelling and language development may be easily adapted to specific lessons or classroom functions. The arrival of a class pet hamster or the filling out of job application forms may be the vehicle for the development of specific language activities (not to mention the knowledge gained about the care and feeding of hamsters or the function of a well–filled-out job application).

Of greatest concern here is not the particular method or presentation of these language activities, but that they not be left out of the curriculum. In the day-to-day calendar of school events, it is often easy to let a particular subject area go unnoticed or at least unattended for some more "important" activity or function. The omission of these academic areas, however, is undefensible. They should be a part of the curriculum at appropriate levels of ability and comprehension for all children at the elementary school level.

A final word here about the language arts area of the curriculum concerns the topic of writing. Many children with physical disabilities will be unable to execute penmanship and writing skills at legible levels. An inability to control both fine and gross motor movements, an inability to grasp and release writing implements, and problems in the control of the writing surface may all combine to produce less than a standard "Palmer Method" product. Several techniques may be used to develop writing implements for children who have difficulty manipulating standard writing materials (Compton and Bigge, 1977). These include the use of hand splints or adapted pencils, pens, crayons, or felt markers. The development and use of these implements or techniques may be in conjunction with activities under the direction of the occupational therapist and may, in fact, be part of the treatment program for the child.

It is important to note that perhaps the main concern for the teacher is to be sensitive to a product that may be faulty and inexact. Expectations for legible penmanship by either the teacher of the child may be unrealistic and frustrating. Although attempts should be made to provide and encourage handwriting skills where physically practical, there may come a time for alternative methods to be explored. The use of the typewriter, with or without keyboard templates, should be encouraged at all grade levels as a substitute for handwritten communications. Typing is an alternative to writing that can be both practical and personally rewarding. The development of typing skills should enhance the overall production of school work and other written communications for the child who is capable of manipulating the keyboard, carriage return, and so on.

Science. The science area of the curriculum should not fall into the realm of "the last minute" or "only if there is nothing else to do and all the movies in the school are being used by someone else" category. Science instruction can be adapted so that all the children in a class are able to participate at either a passive or active level. The ability to observe and/or conduct simple desk or lap experiments, to question, state hypotheses, and determine validity of action are possible and exciting avenues of learning for the child with a physical disability.

> The disabled child requires materials which he may manipulate, which will allow practice in observation, which will develop confidence in his abilities, which will provide practice in working cooperatively with others, and which will give him practice in self-directed activities that require the use of imagination and thought. The most important task the physically disabled child must accomplish is that he must come to see himself as a person able to think and create for himself. (Nemarich and Velleman, 1969 p. 25)

Social studies. Combined within the content area known as social studies are the subjects of history, current events, and the government and institutions of the community. If the eventual goal is to integrate the child with a physical disability into the world of the able-bodied, knowledge of that world must be a part of the school curriculum. For children with disabilities interaction with the outside world is often very limited—to the immediate family, the school, the clinic, the hospital, and the neighborhood. Within each of these places there is space for a rich and varied sense of belonging and understanding, but this sense is limited when these places are compared to the wider world in which they exist. Every effort should be made to bring to the child and to take the child with a disability into those areas of community life and knowledge where the child may be accepted as a participant and viable member. Until recently special education has meant isolation from the social, political, and educational frontiers of societal membership. With the withdrawal and breaking down of social and physical barriers throughout the nation, however, children with physical disabilities can no longer be expected to be satisfied with the isolated existence of the special school, with special categorization, or with condescension by others. The teacher and school must become responsible for educating not only the child but also the community about the benefits of mutual participation and interaction.

Participation in the community must be preceded by a knowledge of the components of the community, including its background, history, and current status of functioning. This learning must be purposeful and planned—a visit to the local post office or newspaper plant must be more than just a field trip. As much as any part of the total school curriculum, this area of social studies may well be the foundation for successful participation in the world outside of the class, school, and home.

Art, music, and physical education/recreation. Although the areas of art, music, and physical education/recreation may not be academic in nature, they are nevertheless important to the total education of children with physical disabilities. Participation in these activities will enhance the overall development of the child and may also provide a background of experiences that may be used during leisure time at home and as the child becomes older and more active in the community. The use of leisure time in a satisfying way is a skill that should be fostered and treated as a serious topic in the school curriculum.

If any implicit or explicit dictum is offered regarding instruction in these three areas of the school curriculum, the following points should probably be most strongly emphasized because of the uncertainty often accompanying these areas:

1. Neither the teacher nor the student need be an artist or have any particular talent in artistic pursuits to have a rewarding artistic experience in the classroom.
2. Neither the teacher nor the student need be a musician or have any particular talent in music to have a good musical experience in the classroom.
3. Neither the teacher nor the student need be a physical education or recreational specialist to have a good physical education or recreational experience in the classroom.

Once the above recognition of nonspecific talent is dealt with, the teacher and children can learn to participate in these activities in a meaningful and enjoyable way. This is not to suggest that a person with talent and creative ability or one who is trained in one or all of these areas is not a boon to the class. Indeed, the teacher who can draw other than a stick figure or play the piano or guitar or who is trained in the development of adaptive physical education or recreational therapy will be able to put this personal competence to good use in the class or school program.

ART. The implication of participation in art activities is the development of a product. When considered in this light, it is not surprising that art activities have been less than appealing to many persons, particularly those with physical disabilities. The point to be made is that art activities should not necessarily be directed toward the completion of a specific product for which a model has been provided or expected. To overcome this comparative mode of activity, it might be better to think of art activities in the class as "messing with media." In many instances, messing with media becomes the end in and of itself: an experience in manipulating materials and objects. This experiencing of media mixing and manipulation can be both satisfying and productive—productive in the sense that children have a feeling of accomplishment without having to measure up to a particular standard. There is something wrong with an art lesson that produces 16 identical turkeys with which to decorate the classroom at Thanksgiving time or that has a high failure rate because the children's turkey feathers are not pasted on in the same order as the teacher's or are not of the accepted color. (Is there something wrong with pink, green, and purple polka-dotted turkey feathers?)

For the child with a physical disability, a paintbrush may be an unsatisfactory tool for painting, much as a pencil may be an unacceptable writing implement. Adaptations are numerous and can be just as productive and fun as more traditional paint spreaders. Big brushes (3 and 4 inches wide) with big handles or paint rollers may spread paint effectively and offer a sense of accomplishment for the child with severe physical and gross motor impairment. Finger painting, as well as toe, elbow, arm, leg, and chin painting, can also be fun if just a bit messy (Alkema, 1967; Harper, 1966). Neither the teacher nor the child should be terribly concerned about creating a mess while engaging in art activities. Child, teacher, clothes, and wheelchairs can be cleaned!

One of the best types of media for children to work with is clay or other molding material. Clay is effective because of its ability to be fired and preserved in a variety of shapes and colors to make handprints, plaques, and other highly valued objects such as dishes or plates. Because of its ease in usage, however, a good alternative to clay may be molding dough. The following recipe can be followed by children and adults alike, and the resulting dough used repeatedly if stored between uses in an airtight container. Different coloring may be added as desired: a batch of orange and a batch of black molding dough may be used at Halloween for pumpkins, witches, and hobgoblins.

Mix three 1-pound cans of flour with three fourths of a 1-pound coffee can of salt. Add tempera paint to the dry mixture or food coloring to three fourths of a cup of liquid salad oil. Mix the oil with 1 quart warm water; mix with the dry ingredients. Keep working past the sticky stage; add flour as needed.

MUSIC. If a teacher can turn the switch on the *on-off* button of a radio or record player, or if the teacher can hum or sing—even off-key—the teacher and children alike can participate in meaningful music activities in the classroom. Music activities can readily and easily be made a part of the other curriculum content areas, such as history, reading, language, mathematics, and current events. The listening to music and the participation in the many forms of music can be a rewarding experience.

Children should be provided with a variety of musical experiences. Personal expression, music appreciation, and the benefits of participation may be gained from singing or listening to music, participating in a rhythm band, making instruments, or belonging to a school chorus or band. Rather than becoming an activity that one has to engage in for the spring concert or open house, music can, and should, be a part of every school day, even if it involves no more than the humming of a favorite tune or 5 minutes of listening to a favorite disc jockey on the radio during a recess period.

PHYSICAL EDUCATION/RECREATION. This area of the school curriculum is one of those most specifically related to the physical characteristics of the child with a disability. The physical limitations and those that are psychologically imposed on the individual may restrict, and in many instances forbid participation in the physical activities, sports, and recreational facilities of the community. This is an area in which the obviousness of disability forces a reacknowledgement by the individual of the limitations imposed by the disability. For the child who may be able to function on an intellectual or scholastic plane that is competitive with able-bodied peers, physical participation in sports or games may be relegated to passive score keeping. For the adult with a disability, restrictions on participation in public recreational facilities may be present in the form of architectural barriers, inconvenience in utilizing public attractions, and poor planning or only lip service to a public statement of accommodations for the handicapped. A case in point for the latter instance is the not-unusual provision of space for wheelchair patrons at spectator events but the lack of provision of accommodations for able-bodied friends to accompany them.

Although there are many problems and barriers that may impede participation in physical education or recreational activities, this is no reason for striking these activities from the lives of those with physical disabilities. Prime considerations for the teacher include the need for a thorough understanding of the requirements of the activity, the evaluation and recommendation of a physician for the child's participation in a particular activity or set of activities, and *the inclination of the child to participate*. There are many of us who would rather be bird watchers than long-distance runners; there are many of us who prefer to watch the ball game from the stands rather than play the game in the community park. Choice in participation is as important for the individual with a disability as it is for one without a disability.

Many children with physical disabilities may need to be taught to play. This is not in reference to playing a specific game; they need to be taught to play, to enjoy themselves in activities that are fun. Many children, because of their disabilities or because of the restrictions placed on them by the family and others, may have limited manipulation of play forms. In addition, instruction in physical education activities for fun and learning and instruction in how to utilize public recreational facilities may need to be a specific part of the curriculum. Public recreational facilities are beginning to provide accommodations for those with physical disabilities with the removal of architectural barriers, the provision of adapted bathroom facilities, and the encouragement of participation through advertising.

Implications for children with multiple disabilities

By now, it should be apparent that there is no such thing as a standard curriculum for children with physical disabilities. There is, likewise, no standard method or teaching technique that is appropriate across the board for these children. Where possible, children with physical disabilities should be provided the same opportunity to learn the same curriculum in the same manner as their able-bodied peers. Where this is not possible, provisions must be made to develop a curriculum that is individual specific. This is the reason for existence of special education for those with disabilities. It is impossible to teach reading if visual perceptual difficulties are ignored. It is impossible and irresponsible to teach the history of the western world when retardation prevents the individual from conceptualizing past or future events outside of a very limited time frame.

The curriculum for children with multiple disabilities will change and vary just as the curriculum changes and varies for children who do not have this multiplicity of problems. It is impossible to prescribe or recommend a means for selecting a particular curriculum; there are simply too many variables. What are the multiple disabilities present (mental retardation, perceptual disorders, language and speech disorders, emotional or personal problems)? How severe and to what degree do these conditions impair learning? These questions and literally thousands more need to be asked about each child. For some children who come to school with several disabilities at severe levels of involvement, the curriculum may be centered around the child's acceptance of being in school or of being separated from his/her mother for the first time. Learning to socialize, to eat foods that may be new or strange, or to be fed by someone other than a parent may form the basis of the curriculum for the child with multiple disabilities. It seems little wonder that these children learn at all, let alone when they are confronted with the many strange and often frightening requirements of school.

As these children learn to participate in the school setting, the curriculum changes with the skills and knowledge acquired from purposeful lessons and incidental learning of the environment. Such changes include more formalized means of communication between the teacher and child, and instruction concerning the characteristics and requirements of the environment. These manipulative exercises may later advance to instruction in the more academic skills at levels appropriate for the child's level of functioning. The teacher cannot make assumptions about either what has gone on before the child has reached the classroom or what will occur in the life of the child after leaving the class. Such educational assumptions of function, past or future, are without merit.

Even for children with multiple disabilities, the teacher has the responsibility to develop in the learner the greatest sense of personal freedom and dignity possible, coupled with the greatest amount of independence training possible for eventual adulthood. The presence of multiple disabilities makes the task more difficult and the steps of advancement smaller, but the sense of accomplishment is no less important.

Psychosocial aspects of the school

Reading and writing aren't everything! Just as there are parties, dances, field trips, spring festivals, school-sponsored Girl Scout and Boy Scout troops, paper drives, and school carnivals in the schools and classes for able-bodied children, so should these activities be part of the program for children with physical disabilities attending special schools and classes. And so should these same activities be made available for participation by children with disabilities who are enrolled in schools with their able-bodied peers.

Opportunities for participation in a wide range of activities need to be made available to the child. Children who are denied participation in activities that engender and enhance the development of the total person through social interactions are restrained from developing a unique part of their own individuality. The building of a wall around people and social functions that excludes others creates a barrier as effective as a barbed wire fence. This barrier affects the feelings a person has about the self and the self in relation to others.

A program devoid of the influences in life that affect emotional well-being can become mechanistic and purposeless. For children whose capacity for manipulating language forms or numerical equations is limited, it may be more beneficial to develop a program that has either a specific emotional growth affective component or a combination of the cognitive and affective components of learning as an integrated whole. Because of a background of failure to succeed, criticism of performance, or devaluation of the self from outside sources and internal forces, children need to be taught that they have control over how they feel—how they value themselves and others—and that they can exert a level of control over a world in which they have previously been manipulated and directed.

Children can learn to feel good about themselves even though they may be wheelchair bound. Children can learn to establish and promote a feeling of worth and importance even though they may be unable to produce intelligible speech. These traits can be developed without the need for manipulation of pencils or books. Simon and O'Rourke (1977) have suggested a variety of exercises to help children establish a sense of their own value and produce an affective tone that will make their interactions with others more stimulating and rewarding. What seems to be of most importance is the realization that "the locus of valuing must come from within the person" (p. 56). There can be little doubt that the feeling of having control and value when there may not have been a previous opportunity for such a feeling would be of significant importance to an individual.

Role of the parents

The parents of the child with a physical disability have the same concerns about their child's growing years as parents of able-bodied children. In addition, they may be confronted and sometimes overwhelmed by a vast array of situations and problems unique to their family and/or the disability of their child. In no implied order of importance, the following questions only begins to touch the surface of parental concerns:

Should we, or can we, have other children?

Do we treat this child like our other children?

How will we pay for all the extras that are needed?

Should we send the child to a regular school, a special school, or a residential school? What is best for our child? For us?

Where can we get clothing that will fit around the braces and not wear out so fast? Are there special patterns available to make the special clothes that are needed?

How long will we have to fix special foods or feed the child?

What will happen to our child when we are dead? Can we get insurance? Where? How much? What kind?

Will it be possible for us to have an active social life? How can we provide a social life for our child when friends live so far away?

Who will sit with our child when we go to the movies or try to take a weekend trip by ourselves?

Does therapy do any good?

How will we be able to confront our child's death?

Do other parents share our feelings or problems? Are we alone?

What does the future hold for us? For me? For our child?

Why did this happen to me—to us? Will our lives ever be normal?

There is, of course, no single correct answer to any of these questions. The parents deal with the life of their child in the manner in which they individually and together are capable of at the moment. They make adjustments to their lives that seem best for all concerned at any given time and place. On the other hand, they make mistakes that may be painfully obvious to others or to themselves at a more distant time.

The parents may choose from a variety of avenues of involvement in the life of their child. Parent groups at schools, as well as agencies, are often available to help with the problems facing parents. The parents may immerse themselves in extraordinary care of their child, and they may volunteer their time to help and benefit other parents; or they may choose simply to be left alone to do whatever they think is best without the outside influence of others and without their participation in outside activities. Some parents do too much; some do too little. It is too easy to be judged and too easy to judge others.

HIGH SCHOOL YEARS

What characterizes the high school years? The movement from childhood to adolescence and emerging adulthood, the developing sense of independence, the preparation for the move into postschool activities, the challenge of higher levels of academic functioning, the responsibilities of a new status of being old enough to participate in some activities but not old enough to participate in others are all included. Adolescent growth and development, when put into the perspective of the person with a physical disability, calls for a sense of urgency in the understanding of problems that may be confronted when high school is over.

For some, the final chapter in formal education will occur during the high school years; for others these years will be used for the development of skills that will see them into and through college, employment, and/or home and family management. High school students with physical disabilities soon become faced with choices that will influence the patterns of life in the postschool years. For students who are academically inclined or who are clearly in pursuit of a professional or occupational goal, these are years for study in preparation for college. For students whose work potential or professional goal setting may be limited because of real or imagined obstacles imposed by the disability, the high school years may be ones of fear, frustration, and loss.

High school programs of study must be able to offer a full range of curricular and extracurricular activities for students with physical disabilities. Students who plan to attend an institution of higher learning will need course work through the various academic departments that will provide the prerequisites for admission into college. Students who plan to work after high school will need a program of work training and skill development through work study and on- and off-campus job training to aid in successful work placement in both the sheltered and competitive employment markets. The curriculum should be able to provide all students with disabilities an opportunity to function in the society and environment in as successful a manner as possible.

Bachmann (1971) conducted a follow-up study of graduates from high school programs for disabled students and brought to light some devastating stastistics: of 167 graduates of special programs studied, only 27 were effectively employed; the overwhelming majority of the graduates depended on television for their contact with the world outside of their homes.

What alternatives should be made available for students with physical disabilities in high school so that their postschool lives are not reduced to the limits of the home and television? In the exploration of alternatives for curriculum development and experiences that will better prepare students for independent adult living, caution needs to be taken so that life goals and functioning are not imposed on students "for their own good." This imposition represents responsibility that does not belong to those in a position to offer training or life alternatives. In developing a curriculum, special educators need to ask themselves questions concerning the appropriateness of this curriculum for the students who will be participating in the program:

Is the traditional academic program an appropriate vehicle for participation in the sphere of life that will be available to the student with a disability?

What are the alternatives to academic areas of preparation?

What are the major problems that will be confronting the student on leaving high school? Do these problems include work, independent living, social and sexual relations, transportation, and economic considerations?

How can students with disabilities best be prepared so that the hours and days in their lives do not revolve around television as their sole link with the world?

What are the functional needs of the individual who must live in a confined world?

What is the educator's responsibility to students in his/her care? Too often, a teacher's concern is directed toward a particular class or grade level; he/she hardly acknowledges what lies ahead for the students. It is not unusual to find that a teacher of kindergarten-aged children with disabilities is shocked when forced to consciously acknowledge that these children will grow up to be adults with disabilities. Although children move on to other teachers, the disability, in most instances, remains.

One answer to these questions has been proposed in the form of a program to prepare high school graduates for participation in the society that will soon surround them: the life experience program (Howard and Bigge, 1977). This alternative program consists of specifically teaching daily living skills that will be useful in reducing the barriers to independent functioning in as wide a social context as possible. The life experience program includes indentification of the numerous daily living experiences that are, or will be, part of the student's greater social environment (experiences involving the use of public transportation, restrooms, and telephones, and the facilities offered in stores, restaurants, banks, and other retail and service-oriented businesses), a task analysis of the skills necessary for carrying out these experiences, and the hierarchical arrangement of the skills identified from the task analysis. This is followed by pretesting to determine the student's present level of functioning, participation in the actual setting, and post-testing to determine the new skill attainment level.

Extracurricular activities

In addition to the activities that provide the instructional milieu of the high school, there are functions that give a wider meaning to schooling for the student:

school dances, student government, membership in clubs and service organizations, sports activities and homecoming weekend, school plays, and yearbook activities. Many students participate in one or more of these activities, depending on their interests and personalities. Others choose not to participate according to their own particular inclinations. The point to be made here is that participation in these activities, whether from a spectator's level or from an active participant's level, should be the choice of the student. Participation on the football squad is not feasible for the wheelchair-bound student. On the other hand, the possibility of participation on a wheelchair basketball, swimming, or gymnastics team may not be out of the question. And is there any reason why a student on crutches should not try out for cheerleader, be sponsored as homecoming queen, or take pictures for the high school yearbook?

If the above activities are an important part of the lives of high school students, the one that probably most signifies the coming of age or a sense of emerging independence is that of learning to drive a car and obtaining that holy writ, a driver's license. Driver's education and special equipment are now available to provide high school–aged students with physical disabilities the skills necessary to safely and properly drive a car. The standard power equipment options available on most cars (power brakes, power steering, automatic transmission, and so on) can be supplemented with such devices as hand controls for the accelerator and brakes, left-sided gearshift levers, and automatic door openers. Once driving skill has been developed, the student must then contend with the additional problems of acquiring insurance at a reasonable cost, being able to absorb the costs of buying a car and outfitting it with the special equipment that may be needed, and providing maintenance and upkeep of the car. The dream of ownership and the love affair with the car by a teenager is ever present, and many persons with disabilities are now driving and experiencing a level of travel independence not known in the past.

Implications for students with multiple disabilities

The high school student with multiple disabilities may have the same needs in relation to learning that were expressed in the elementary school years. The imposition of retardation, perceptual disorders, or of multiple physical disabilities will still need to be taken into consideration in both the curriculum and the methods of presentation. Concern needs to be directed at this point toward the challenges that the immediate future holds for the student on completion of high school and toward the goals that can be established for long-range adult living.

Utilization of a special curriculum such as the life experience program mentioned previously may be of some benefit to students with multiple disabilities, as may the development of work-training skills or skills that may be employed by the student whose future may not include work. Arts and crafts activities that may be adapted to suit the abilities and interests of the person with multiple disabilities may be explored and developed. The ability to use the telephone may also be practiced so that communication with friends may be maintained beyond the school environment.

It is a fact that not all persons with physical disabilities or multiple disabilities will be able to live independently, drive a car, hold a job, or maintain a home or family. To suggest that this is so would be to foster an illusion. To suggest that there can be dignity and purpose in one's life without these activities is, however, well within reason. Alternatives to home living need to be explored. Knowledge in the availability of live-in attendants and aides should be part of the curriculum of the high school student, as should knowledge concerning financial support available through various public and private agencies. Student projects in high school can be directed toward finding resources that will be beneficial in postschool life: transportation systems, meal preparation services, home management services, health services, and so on.

If the schools maintain the position of the need to develop students to the fullest extent possible for admission into independent adult society, then this commitment must extend to all levels of education and to all persons with disabilities. Failure to identify and implement a curriculum for those with multiple disabilities is less than no commitment to education at all.

Role of the parents

The parents of the high school student with a physical disability are confronted with problems similar to the ones they confronted in earlier years. Now they must also contend with problems associated with the movement of their child into adolescence and early adulthood and with the striving and desire for independence from the nest. Many high school students with physical disabilities will meet with frustrations and failures, and parents will need to be able to provide a level of comfort and support that extends beyond the scope of sympathy and into the realm of understanding. They will need to understand their child's anger at not being invited to a dance, his/her frustration and embarrassment at still needing to be toileted by a parent, and the rejection their child suffers at the hands of others as he/she begins to explore participation in the world of adulthood.

The parents may need to confront some of their own anxieties as they begin to look again into the future. What will become of the child? What will become of the parents? Such questions as how and where the child will live and what will be the parents' responsibility in that living space need to be asked. What should be told about sex, sexual functioning, and sexuality? Is family planning information important? What should be told about family planning, and when? Answers to these questions can hardly ever be answered once and for all. Adjustments to the disability—to the facts that their child has a disability and that they are the parents of a child with a disability—need to be made again and again as the child changes. Once made, adjustments and life decisions do not last forever; they need to be reexamined and reassessed as new and changing conditions are imposed on the family unit.

In some instances, the flight of their child from the nest is particularly difficult for the parents of a child with a disability. When the majority of the life space of a parent has been directed toward the care of the child, the parents may feel a great sense of loss and abandonment when that care is no longer needed or at least not with the same intensity as before. On the other hand, the parents may be frustrated at the lack of independence that is afforded other parents when their children leave home. For parents who must maintain a physical and emotional care-giving relationship with their child into adulthood, a feeling of anger and guilt may settle in with the realization that the end is not yet in sight.

Parenting is not easy, but there are rewards as well as sacrifices. There are accomplishments as well as setbacks. Quite simply, the overriding need is love.

SUMMARY

This chapter has provided information regarding the curriculum and instruction that may be used with children with physical disabilities from the preschool years through high school. It has been indicated that there is no specific curriculum or methodology that may be employed in teaching children with disabilities. Some of the implications of teaching children with multiple disabilities have been explored, as have some of the extracurricular activities that are associated with the school years.

A curriculum should be as individual specific as need be to develop the child to the fullest extent possible. The methods used should be eclectic and within the realm of physical safety and comfort. Within this realm, there should not be an avoidance of content because of the presence of the disability in the student; rather the content should be adapted to meet the learning needs of the student for independent functioning in adult life.

REFERENCES

Alkema, C. Implications of art for the handicapped child; out of the classroom. *Exceptional Children,* 1967, *33,* 433-434.

Bachmann, W. H. *Influence of selected variables upon economic adaptation of orthopedically handicapped and other health impaired.* Unpublished doctoral dissertation, University of the Pacific, 1971.

Compton, C., and Bigge, J. Academics. In J. Bigge and P. A. O'Donnell (Eds.), *Teaching individuals with physical and multiple disabilities.* Columbus, Ohio: Charles E. Merrill Publishing Co., 1977.

Connor, F. P. The education of children with crippling and chronic medical conditions. In W. M. Cruickshank and G. O. Johnson (Eds.), *Education of exceptional children and youth (3rd ed.).* Englewood Cliffs, N.J.: Prentice-Hall, Inc., 1975.

Developmentally Delayed Infant Education Project (The). *Infant stimulation curriculum.* Columbus, Ohio: The Nisonger Center for Mental Retardation and Developmental Disabilities, The Ohio State University.

Dorward, B. *Teaching aids and toys for handicapped children.* Reston, Va.: The Council for Exceptional Children, 1960.

Eliason, C. F., and Jenkins, L. T. *A practical guide to early childhood curriculum.* St. Louis: The C. V. Mosby Co., 1977.

Ellis, N. E., and Cross, L. (Eds). *Planning programs for early education of the handicapped.* New York: Walker and Co., 1977.

Finnie, N. R. *Handling the young cerebral palsied child at home (2nd ed.).* New York: E. P. Dutton & Co., Inc., 1975.

Harper, G. Toe painting—a special education project, out of the classroom. *Exceptional Children,* 1966, *33,* 123-124.

Howard, R., and Bigge, J. Life experiencing programming. In J. Bigge and P. A. O'Donnell

(Eds.), *Teaching individuals with physical and multiple disabilities*. Columbus, Ohio: Charles E. Merrill Publishing Co., 1977.

Koontz, C. W. *Koontz child developmental program training activities for the first 48 months*. Los Angeles: Western Psychological Services, 1974.

Meier, J. H. Screening, assessment, and intervention for young children at developmental risk. In T. D. Tjossem (Ed.), *Intervention strategies for high risk infants and young children*. Baltimore: University Park Press, 1976.

Myers, C. (Ed.), *The live oak curriculum: a guide to preschool planning in the heterogeneous classroom*. Piedmont, Calif.: Alpha Plus Corp., Circle Preschool, 1977.

Nemarich, S. P., and Velleman, R. A. *The modification of educational equipment and for maximum utilization by physically disabled persons*. Albertson, N.Y.: Human Resources Center, 1969.

Quick, A. D., and Campbell, A. A. *Lesson plans for enhancing preschool developmental progress*. Dubuque, Iowa: Kendall/Hunt Publishing Co., 1976.

Segal, M. M. *From birth to one year*. Fort Lauderdale, Fla.: Nova University, 1974.

Segal, M. M., and Adcock, D. *From one to two years*. Fort Lauderdale, Fla.: Nova University.

Simon, S. B., and O'Rourke, R. D. *Developing values with exceptional children*. Englewood Cliffs, N.J.: Prentice-Hall, Inc., 1977.

Tjossem, T. D. *Intervention strategies for high risk infants and young children*. Baltimore: University Park Press, 1976.

Wabash Center for the Mentally Retarded, Inc. *Guide to early developmental training*. Boston: Allyn & Bacon, Inc., 1977.

8 Postschool and adult alternatives

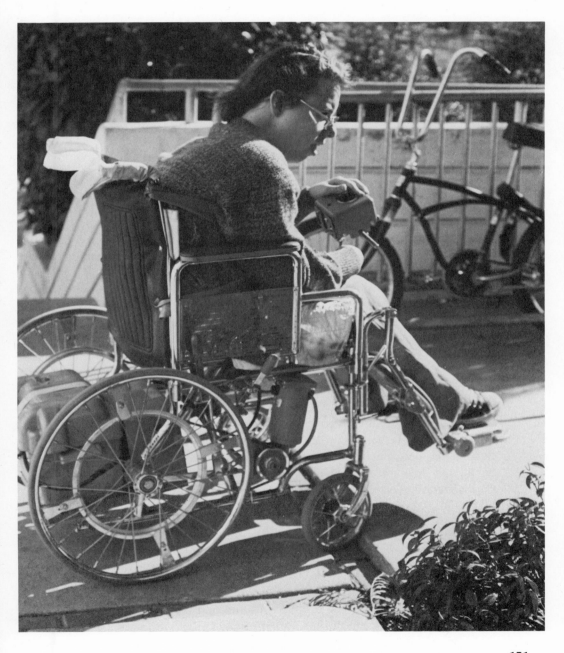

Children with physical disabilities grow up and become adults with physical disabilities. Although this may appear on the surface to be a gross oversimplification, it is nevertheless a point that many teachers fail to acknowledge. It is most easy to concentrate on the day-to-day requirements of the third grade classroom and lose sight of the end product of the school system: the independently functioning adult. This nearsighted approach to educational provisions and services for children with disabilities may occur for a variety of reasons: assumptions made about the future functioning of an individual student based on present behavior, school achievement, and physical characteristics; a lack of knowledge—or worse, a lack of concern—about the future adult world of school-aged children; and the assumption that since the adult with a disability is more or less absorbed into society, the educational system has done its job in providing adequate preparation for emergence into that arena. It might be instructive for teachers to ask themselves and others, "What will happen to the students in my class 10 years from now?" Or, "What are the students I taught 10 years ago doing today?"

The follow-up studies of school graduates are numerous; the findings, disastrous! Generally, the studies have found that students who have completed or taken part in special education programs are unemployed or underemployed; they lack independent living opportunities or skills; and they do not have available or do not participate in the social and recreational opportunities considered by the able-bodied majority to be consistent with a "full life" or a "successful status" (Bachmann, 1971; Brieland, 1967; Klapper and Birch, 1966; Olshansky and Beach, 1975; Vogel, 1975). Has education done its job? Have we, as educators, fulfilled our commitments?

Adults with physical disabilities are coming out of the closet. Those with disabilities are the most conscious of their lack of preparation for participation in the world of the able-bodied, and they are beginning to become a force that must be recognized and dealt with. The civil rights movement has reached a level of recognition and respect that today encompasses those with disabilities. Legislation has guaranteed the right to education for all handicapped children; legislation has also been enacted eliminating the denial of jobs based solely on disability; barrier-free environments are being demanded and acquired because of legislation and the funding requirements for construction and manufacture. The elimination of these barriers to independent existence is a process that Park (1975) has described as normalization. According to Park, the elements of normalization are:

> (1) Righting the wrongs of the past. (2) Bringing the handicapped back into the mainstream of society. (3) Developing the "normal" as a risk process that involves the elimination of the "sanitized life" and substituting for it the possibility of failure as well as the possibility of greater rewards." (p. 108)

The remainder of this chapter is presented in a format unlike that of the rest of this book. Through the cooperation and permission of *The Independent,* a series of articles is presented from the spring 1977 issue of this journal that reflect some of the concerns of the independent adult. *The Independent* is published quarterly by the Center for Independent Living, Inc. (CIL), a nonprofit organization providing services for those with disabilities and/or who are blind. The subjects dealt with in the articles presented here include the political force that those with disabilities can exert, the problem of public transportation accessibility, the self-care needs of the adult, the financial needs of and advocacy support for those with disabilities, personal needs in relation to the development of the child with a disability as expressed from the viewpoint of the adult with a disability, and sexuality and sexual functioning as described by a young man with a disability. The final article is a parody that strips away the fiction and sighs at the truth.

The first article addresses the issue of how persons with disabilities are perceived. Are they, as a group, subject to protection for their own good? Or are they subject to the same conditions for successful living and employment as others?

YOU CAN FIGHT CITY HALL!
by Ken Stein

In a landmark ruling on Tuesday, May 18, the Berkeley City Council overturned a Berkeley Fire Department order which would have forced CIL's computer training project out of its present quarters. The project is located on the

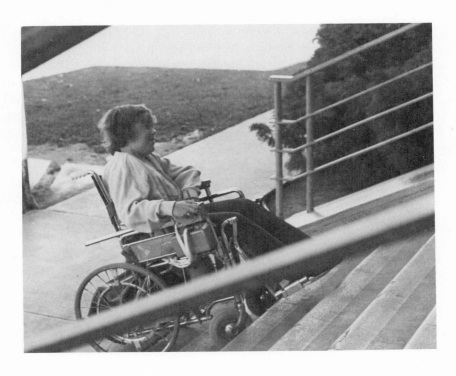

fourth floor of a building in downtown Berkeley. Speaking for CIL at the hearing, Deputy Director Judy Heumann said that "as disabled individuals we have worked very hard to remove from the public the image of persons with disabilities as being hopeless, helpless cripples. Yet the fire department contends that if there are more than five or six persons who are labeled by the state as being non-ambulatory then the code which must be applied is that which is applicable to hospitals and other institutions. The implication once again is that we are unable to take responsibility for ourselves."

CIL could have moved. However, rather than yielding to the eviction order, CIL began lobbying the City Council. This effort extended over a two month period. Throughout these meetings we stressed that our concern was for the safety of all people. We argued effectively that if the building was unsafe for persons with visible disabilities, then it was unsafe for all people and should be shut down entirely.

CIL also worked with and received letters of support from the State Council on Developmental Disabilities, HEW's Office of Civil Rights and the National Center on Law and the Handicapped. The consensus among these agencies was that a ruling against the Center would have extremely negative repercussions for the disabled population throughout the country.

We contended that such a negative precedent would have perpetuated cases of discrimination in housing, education, and independent living. The ruling could easily have led to forced evacuation of thousands of Berkeley's disabled people living above the ground floors of buildings.

At the May 18 meeting, there were more than 100 representatives from CIL. We also received strong community support at the hearing from Community Services United, a coalition of over 20 community agencies.

The fire department contended that the building lacked "adequate and safe exiting designed for use by non-ambulatory and handicapped persons." Harvey Clausen, the Deputy State Fire Marshall, said that "it is not the intent of the fire authorities to interfere with any program designed to assist handicapped people to assume self-reliance; rather, it was their intent to assist them in this endeavor by maintaining a safe environment for them so that this goal may be met."

In rejecting the order, Berkeley's Major Widener said, "To me, the critical point is that we just can't make every building totally safe for everybody. If a person breaks a foot and they're in a building, then they're not as ambulatory as someone else. I've been impressed by the statement by people at CIL that they feel they're being discriminated against in that we're so concerned about their safety that we're applying standards to them that we really don't apply to other people."

At the meeting, the City Council also rejected a motion to appoint a committee to establish standards relating to commercial and residential occupancy by people with disabilities. In speaking to the motion, Councilwoman Hone said that "We should ask the City Manager informally to continue to review our buildings to insure that buildings are built safely for everyone of every age. But I think that anything that we would do as a council appointed committee would begin to penalize people in terms of whether buildings would be available to them. The thrust of the motion may run counter to what most of us have come to feel—that special standards are restrictive to people living a full life." In her closing statement, Councilwoman Hancock said, "I feel very good about what we did tonight. I think we indicated that we have set a very good precedent by refusing to set a precedent that would limit in any way the rights of disabled people to live and work throughout this city. I think we have also indicated a concern to keep buildings safe for all human beings and that we will single out no category of persons for particular treatment that would exclude them from living and working in certain places."

The City Council's ruling applies only to Berkeley, but we believe it has far-reaching implications. There have been numerous pieces of legislation passed which protect the rights of citizens with disabilities. Had the fire department prevailed, the intent of these laws would have been greatly undermined. By refusing to yield, CIL was able to bring about a ruling demonstrating that persons with disabilities must be treated equally and will no longer accept being segregated from their communities.

What are the limits imposed on a person who is wheelchair bound and unable to travel freely in the environment? Is the answer as simple as the restriction of movement from point A to point B? Although more public transportation facilities are adapting to the needs of those with disabilities, there are still a variety of limitations that need to be confronted to enable these individuals to have more complete freedom of travel.

WHY DISABLED PEOPLE DO NOT USE BART (TECHNICALLY ACCESSIBLE)
by Hale Zukas

In June of 1973 the Bay Area Rapid Transit System (BART) began limited operation. This modern system was designed to be accessible to disabled persons. Whether it serves the disabled population is a question that must take notice of psychological barriers to its use.

A person's "range of mobility" is the area in which he perceives himself as being able to travel as a matter of course. The expansion of this range depends upon his awareness of travel needs, as well as upon the availability of new means of transportation.

It follows that if a person is physically disabled, the development of his range of mobility has probably been arrested at an early stage, since many means of transportation are closed to him. Consequently, he is unlikely to have considered destinations of the sort that BART is intended to reach. The fact that BART makes it easier to get to an office, store or place of entertainment 15 or 20 miles away does not mean anything to someone who is homebound because he has no way of getting up or down the steps to his place of residence. If such a person were asked where he would go if he could, he is likely to say he would go outside to get some sun and perhaps go around his immediate neighborhood. It is even conceivable that he would respond to this question by saying that he could not think of any place he would like to go.

Incredible and pathetic as such a response may seem, it is understandable when viewed in the larger context. People who have been immobile for many years simply have no idea of the impact mobility can have on their lives. (They do not realize, to give just one example, that mobility makes it immensely easier to develop and maintain friendships.) This lack of awareness is not just simple ignorance; it is also a defense mechanism: knowledge of what mobility can mean can only be frustrating to those who are immobile.

That the solution to this problem involves a number of interacting factors is demonstrated by the experience of the Physically Disabled Students' Program (PDSP) at the University of California at Berkeley. The PDSP provides transportation service, using two specially modified vans that have hydraulic lifts, wheelchair lockdowns and raised roofs. The vans are driven by PDSP staff, and the service is provided at no cost to the user. In sum, the service is provided at no cost to the needs of disabled people. Furthermore, the disabled students served by the program are, almost by definition, much more active and better equipped socially than the average disabled person.

It might be expected that under these most favorable conditions a rapid and substantial increase in the level of mobility of a large group of disabled people would occur. Such was not the case, however. Instead, demand grew only gradually, and it was not until a year and a half after their acquisition that the vans began to be utilized fully. Since the nature of the service did not change appreciably in that period, we can conclude that the slow rate of increase in demand was due to lack of client awareness. In other words, time was needed for the travel objectives of the client population to evolve to a level which corresponded to the opportunities offered by the newly available transportation service.

In this context, BART is an even more sophisticated mode of transportation. It is intended to serve those whose range of mobility is already highly developed; those, in other words, who have come to freely use what might be termed "more basic" forms of transportation. Indeed, BART is designed explicitly to rely heavily on such forms of transportation as feeders. But the ability to use a car or bus is needed not only for the pragmatic reason that most people must use a car or bus to reach BART; it is also necessary in the more profound sense: the awareness of travel objectives that BART is useful in reaching is likely to develop only through the use of more basic forms of transportation.

BART is widely noted for its accessibility to the handicapped and, to be sure, it is more accessible than any other major transit system in the country. But it is accessible only in the narrowest sense of the word. One of the primary purposes of this discussion has been to demonstrate that in order to be meaningful for wheelchair travelers, accessibility must be defined in broader terms, going far beyond the installation of elevators or ramps, important as that is. In this larger sense, BART must be considered inaccessible, for as has been shown above, there are still substantial barriers, both practical and psychological, which act to impede the disabled from using the system.

Can a disability be overcome, or can freedom from physical limitation be found to the degree that a measure of independence in living can be achieved? The need to be on one's own, to have the dignity of feeling that there is a level of control over life maintenance, is discussed in the following two articles. Practical suggestions may make the difference between comfort and discomfort, security and insecurity.

MOBILITY IN BED
by Greg Sanders

Perhaps the greatest restriction for severely disabled persons trying to live independently is not their mobility during the day, but their lack of mobility in bed. It is, at best, annoying to depend on an attendant to get out of bed one or more times during the night to turn you, not to mention the financial aspect or the hassle of finding a live-in attendant. Maximizing your mobility in bed requires a lot of effort and imagination, but the benefit of independence curing that half of your life is well worth it.

The key to this mobility is employing either electrical power to compensate for a lack of physical strength or a well planned system of straps and bars which enable you to make the most of the strength you do have. If properly used, an electric hospital bed can perform both of these functions. The combination of the side rails and an overhead trapeze bar with a suspended loop of nylon webbing provides a number of positions which can be used for leverage. For example, if a quadriplegic can swing one wrist up into the suspended loop then slide his other wrist against either a vertical or horizontal bar in the side rail, he can turn himself by lifting with the arm in the loop and pulling with the arm against the rail. When the shoulders are turned in this manner, the momentum will carry the hips and legs through the turn.

Often, a turn like this may cause the legs to spasm up into a bent position. One way to get the legs straight again is to secure a padded strap around the ankles and fasten it to a weight on the floor. Then, pushing the "bed-up" button on an electric bed will raise the bed and pull the legs straight.

For an elaborate system of loops, a "balkan frame" can be placed on top of most hospital beds. Basically, it is a pattern of bars supported four feet or so above the bed. These bars provide a foundation for suspending a number of loops. The additional positions available for leverage significantly help with transferring and general mobility; however, without some imaginative decorating the bars may appear somewhat oppressive.

If the narrow width of a hospital bed crowds your sleeping, it isn't very difficult to adjust the bed to accommodate a larger mattress. The simplest method is to bolt 1 inch sheets of plywood to the frame. If the plywood is cut like the original mattress frame, the bed can still be raised into a sitting position. Similarly, a common bed can be modified to perform most of the functions of a hospital bed. For instance, most medical supply houses sell overhead trapezes which support themselves and can, therefore, be used with any bed. Also, with a little constructive work, side rails can be adapted to most beds, or a few bars or loops can be strategically placed instead of rails.

If lack of physical strength or something else prevents you from turning during the night, there are various mattress supplements which may help your situation; however, every disabled person must be aware of the possibility of pressure sores and be careful about staying in one position too long. The most common mattress supplements which can be purchased from almost any medical supply house are: (1) foam rubber mattress covers, (2) artificial sheepskins, (3) silicone or gel pads for the hips and more sensitive pressure points, and (4) a pulsating mattress. The pulsating mattress is probably the most effective means of avoiding too much pressure on any one area. It consists of a number of pressurized air compartments which routinely open and close, thus, constantly shifting the pressure. They sell for about $125.

After you have developed a method for turning, the other necessities for sustaining yourself independently through the night—like having access to water, etc.—may take awhile to perfect, but should be relatively easy. However, you should always keep in mind the possibility of an accident or emergency and have some way of contacting help if necessary. This can be done as easily as keeping a telephone within reach or using an intercom to connect you with other parts of the house. Wireless intercoms come in many models and begin near $25 for a pair.

FINDING A GOOD ATTENDANT
by Don Berry

An attendant is a person who helps you do things you are physically unable to do yourself. Often these attendants are hard to find. If you live in an area where there is no organization such as the CIL that provides attendant referrals, then the following sources should be utilized in your search:

1. College bulletin boards and placement office.
2. Friends who use attendants.
3. Local newspapers, including college papers.
4. Employment office.
5. Public Health Department.
6. Hospital bulletin boards.

After ads have been placed, people will call for information. Explain your general situation and arrange to meet the person. Do not hire a person sight unseen. The purpose of the interview is to inform the person exactly what the job involves. This includes wages, hours to work, problems that may arise and responsibilities at the job.

If you require an attendant for different times throughout the day, it is helpful to employ more than one person. This eliminates the problem of one person working seven days a week. It is also helpful in an emergency when one person is unable to work.

Some helpful hints in finding and keeping good attendants:

1. Attendants should be paid for the entire time spent on the job. They should also be paid for time spent waiting for the employer.
2. The very minimum of $2/hr. should be paid for every hour worked.
3. Attendants should be paid $3/hr. for all work after midnight, plus transportation costs, in compensation for the late hour and risk involved in travel.
4. Pay on time.
5. Hire only people you feel are qualified to do the job.
6. Don't hire a person if you foresee personality or employment conflicts.
7. Often people looking for attendant work have no experience. Don't be afraid to explain to the person how you need the job done. You know your needs better than anyone else.

Finally, try to pool your attendant information with other disabled people you know. The more contacts you have the better the chance of finding qualified attendants.

The following two articles provide specific suggestions for the acquisition of levels of independence for those with disabilities. The financial means by which life support, dignity, and self-worth may be enjoyed are identified. Although many of the recommendations and suggestions are related to California aid programs, the content of these two articles may well serve as a guide for the investigation of sources in other areas. We all experience a level of dependency for our existence, but much of that dependency may be the result of occupations of our own choosing, life-styles of our own making, and conditions of life that are created as nearly by our own power as possible. Persons with physical disabilities need these same choices and power of command and demand.

PLANS TO ACHIEVE SELF-SUPPORT
by Greg Sanders

A common characteristic of many American public assistance programs is their overwhelming tendency to create lifetime recipients. That is, once individuals become dependent on a system, they are frequently prohibited from accumulating the necessary income, resources, or training to break away from their dependency. Fortunately, the authors of the Supplemental Security Income (SSI) program recognized the problem and attempted to remove this self-perpetuating tendency from the system. Their intent is manifested through the exclusion of any income or property used to meet the occupational goal of an approved plan to achieve self-support. The primary factors in developing and implementing a self-support plan are discussed in this article; however, if more specific information is required, consult the Social Security Administration Claims Manual 12460 through 12470.

Excess income and resources

First, it must be realized that eligibility for SSI is based on need as defined by specific income and resource limitations. Before considering the function of a self-support plan, the basic aspects of income and resource treatment must be understood. "Income" refers to the value of any earnings, pensions, gifts, etc., received in a calendar quarter. Any item of value retained into the following quarter becomes a resource. "Resources" include property, savings, stock bonds, etc. Individuals must not exceed the allowable amount of resources. If they do, the general philosophy is that they should convert the excess resources to cash and use that cash to provide for their needs before receiving public assistance. After the excess has been reduced, the individual will meet the resource limitation and become eligible for aid.

The treatment of income is somewhat different. An applicant/recipient may have excess income and still receive aid, but the amount of excess income will affect the level of benefits received. For the purpose of this article, it is sufficient to understand that income will be excluded from consideration in specific circumstances, or will be considered countable (excess) income. "Excluded income" is available to the applicant/recipient to spend as s/he pleases. It will not affect the level of benefits. "Countable income" is considered to be in excess of the amount necessary to maintain a healthy livelihood and, therefore, reduces the level of benefits. If the benefits are reduced to zero, eligibility ends.

In the event that an applicant/recipient may have excess income or resources, the excess may be applied toward an approved plan for self-support and, thus, become excluded from consideration. Assuming that all excess resources and/or income is applied toward the plan, eligibility will not be jeopardized by the excess and the individual will receive the full benefit level. In short, this provision allows both applicants and recipients of SSI to have any amount of income or resources and still be eligible for full benefits as long as the portion of their income and/or resources which exceeds the normal allowable levels is used toward an approved attempt to become self-supporting.

Guidelines

Of course, there are specific conditions which must be met before the exclusion for a self-support plan will be accepted by the Social Security Administration (SSI); yet, the guidelines are reasonable and easy to deal with. The conditions are:

1. A specific plan to achieve self-support must exist in writing.
2. The plan must be approved by SSA, but SSA will request the Department of Rehabilitation (DR), a state agency for the blind, or the Veteran's Administration to evaluate the vocational feasibility of a plan.
3. The plan must contain specific savings goals and/or planned disbursements for a designated occupational objective, and a specific period of time for achieving it.
4. The plan must provide for the identification and segregation of money and goods, if any, being accumulated and conserved.
5. The plan must be current.
6. The individual must be performing in accordance with the plan.

Implementation of a plan

In the fall of 1976 substantial training in self-support plans was provided to DR staff, and some training to SSA staff. Nonetheless, district offices of SSA and DR will vary in their knowledge of this issue. Furthermore, the understanding of self-support plans may vary among persons within any given district office. Thus, it is to the advantage of an individual attempting to implement a plan to understand the process as well as possible. The following procedure has been used successfully by clients of CIL and should be useful to persons in other areas or states. However, CIL has been fortunate in receiving exceptional cooperation from the SSA and DR district offices. If a problem arises in implementing a specific case, consult the Social Security Administration Claims Manual as mentioned earlier.

First, you must develop the occupational goal of your plan. You may do this yourself or request assistance from a DR counselor. The general guideline for a goal is the purchase of equipment or training necessary to achieve self-support or substantially increase self-sufficiency. Under this flexible guideline, practically any occupational expenditure which will legitimately facilitate an attempt to achieve self-support is acceptable. For example, the goal may be to apply excess income and/or resources to purchase tools, space, or business license for a carpentry profession; or, to pay tuition for a graduate degree; or, perhaps to purchase an adequate vehicle necessary for employment. The primary factor in developing a goal is to relate any purchase to your vocational objective.

After your goal is clear, you must develop a specific written plan. There is no necessary format to follow, simply be sure to include the necessary information:

I. List the income and/or resources to be applied toward the plan. Be specific. When possible, identify an item by bank account number, serial number, license, etc.

II. List all the items to be purchased or accumulated to meet the occupational objective of the plan. Also, list the cost of each item as accurately as possible.

III. Provide a narrative statement discussing exactly why each item to be purchased is necessary for your achievement of self-support. In most cases, the necessity of an item will be clear; thus, the narrative may be very brief.

IV. Outline how the plan will operate. For instance, you may wish to deposit funds in a savings account, then draw from that account to provide a down payment and monthly installments for an item. In this case, state the bank account number and how the payments will be made. Also, state that you will save receipts, etc., to verify all expenditures. Whatever method of operating, the plan you choose must provide a means of identifying all funds and resources and must verify any action you have taken. Also, you must accumulate self-support plan funds separately from all personal savings.

V. State when your goal will be achieved. Initially, the duration of a plan is limited to no longer than 18 months. So draft your original plan for up to 18 months. After the original 18 month period, you may receive an extension of 18 additional months for "good cause." When an extension is approved, you may revise the anticipated date of achievement. Also, the duration of a plan involving education may be up to 48 months. In this case, a second extension of up to 12 months may be requested after the first 18 month extension. When filing a self-support plan you must state an anticipated date for achieving your occupational objective. This date may be revised at any time with DR/SSA approval as long as the maximum duration limit is not exceeded.

Approval of plans

After a plan exists in writing, it must be approved. SSA has the authority to approve or deny a plan, yet will almost always refer vocational evaluation of the plan to DR. Logically, DR is the public agency best suited to evaluate the vocational aspects of disability or blindness and may contribute to the development and implementation of an individual's achievement objective. To be sure, approval of a plan to achieve self-support should not be taken for granted. However, each person will have the opportunity to discuss his or her plan in detail with a DR counselor. Certainly, there is no reason to doubt that a legitimate attempt toward self-support will be approved.

Footwork

Recipients who have a DR counselor should present their written plan to that counselor for approval. Persons who do not have a DR counselor should present their written plan to SSA. The SSA can approve or deny the plan, but will probably refer the individual to DR. For persons without a DR counselor, it may facilitate implementation of a self-support plan if they contact SSA for the referral to DR as opposed to contacting DR first. Also, any person without a DR counselor who desires help in devising a plan may contact SSA for a referral to DR.

After you have discussed the plan with a DR counselor and received a verbal approval of the plan, SSA must be notified. To minimize the possibility of red tape delays, report the existence of your approved plan directly to SSA. You should present SSA your written plan and the name and address of your DR counselor. Then, SSA will send an information exchange form to the DR counselor to verify the approval.

The SSA form for verification of approval is very short, approximately one page. Accordingly, the DR counselor will have to condense information about your plan into short statements. Realizing this, you should be sure that your written plan is clearly stated and, of course, legible. It may facilitate implementation of the plan if you provide the DR counselor with two plans—one detailed narrative plan which the counselor may keep for reference and one copy which briefly outlines the basic facts. Also, SSA will want to know the present status of the plan. To provide this information simply include in the outline of your plan how much income and resources you have set aside to meet your goal and what expenditures, if any, you have presently made toward the goal.

When DR returns the form with the appropriate information and approval, SSA will input the exclusion of income/resources into the SSI system. In some cases, applying the exclusion of income/resources will require a change in the level of benefits, and in other cases a change will not be necessary. For example, a recipient who is receiving full SSI benefits, then begins to receive Social Security Disability Insurance Benefits (SSDI), can exclude the excess income created by the SSDI benefits under a plan to achieve self-support. If the self-support plan begins when the SSDI benefits begin, the individual remains eligible for full Supplemental Security Income (SSI) benefits, and the system continues payments without interruption. Conversely, a person who receives only partial SSI benefits due to a source of excess income (i.e., SSDI benefits) and begins to exclude the excess income under a self-support plan, will become entitled to full SSI benefits. As such, the SSI system must change the monthly payment to the recipient.

When the implementation of a self-support plan requires a change in the payment level, the recipient must be prepared for a brief disruption in aid. With luck, the SSI computer will accept the new programming and begin the correct payment. However, until the programming procedure is refined, it is possible that the computer will issue incorrect payments. If a computer error causes a recipient to be underpaid, SSA will correct the payment. Similarly, if an error causes a recipient to be overpaid, SSA will request the recipient to repay the excess amount. Thus, to prevent additional difficulties, a recipient should maintain an accurate record of all SSI payments immediately following implementation of a plan.

Operation of the plan

When SSA inputs the exclusion for a plan into the system, the plan is placed in a folder and notated to be reviewed one month before the end of the plan. Unless SSA is notified by the recipient or DR that the plan has ended prematurely, the plan will operate until it is reviewed. Since most plans begin with an 18 month duration, the review should occur in the 17th month. At this time, one extension of up to 18 months may be approved if the recipient can show "good cause." Ideally, SSA will review the plan just prior to its termination and inform the recipient of his/her SSI status when the excess income/resources which were excluded under the plan become countable. Yet it is very possible that SSA will be burdened with other red tape and delay this determination. If benefits are incorrectly continued after the end of a plan, any overpayment will be collected by SSA.

If the self-support plan was followed exactly as outlined, the plan will simply be terminated at the end of the specified duration. As the plan ceases to exist, excess income/resources become countable and affect aid accordingly. However, it is important to note that the basic treatment of resources excludes from consideration equipment necessary for self-support. Thus equipment purchased in a plan to achieve self-support will not affect eligibility as long as it remains necessary for employment. (CM 12600-12615).

Revisions

The specified savings and disbursements of a plan may be revised at any time with approval of DR and SSA. Since plans may commonly involve a very lengthy period, it is reasonable that revisions may be necessary to achieve the self-support objective. To implement a revision simply alter the specific written conditions of the plan and submit the request to DR and SSA for approval. It is very important that any change in a self-support plan be promptly reported to SSA and DR for formal approval.

Unsuccessful attempts

It should be clear that this exclusion is provided to encourage an individual to attempt self-support. As such, there is no penalty for failing to meet the objectives of the plan. If a plan is ended prematurely, the income/resources which were excluded for the plan and not applied toward the objective simply become countable in the quarter following the termination of the plan. Similarly, if a plan ends before all the income/resources excluded for the plan are applied toward the occupational objective, the remaining income resources are considered countable in the next quarter. For example, if a plan prematurely ended in March, any income/resources excluded for the plan but not actually applied toward the occupational objective would be considered countable for the quarter beginning in April.

Conclusion

Of course, there are additional considerations for specific cases, but this discussion should provide a basis for implementing a plan to achieve self-support. Before closing the discussion, however, a few random facts which relate to common difficulties should be mentioned.

1. Any income or property may be excluded if applied toward an approved self-support plan. Some persons maintain that this exclusion applies only to income received from employment. They are incorrect.

2. The function of a self-support plan is limited to the exclusion of income or resources as they relate to determining financial "need." Income (specifically, "earned income") is also a criterion in determining "disability" status. A self-support plan cannot exclude income in relationship to disability determination. Despite an 18 month self-support plan, a recipient could lose his or her disability status after a 9 month "Trial Work Period" due to "Substantial Gainful Activity" and, therefore, lose all SSI benefits. (See in the Summer 1975 issue of *The Independent,* "Employment: How it affects SSI.")

3. A plan to achieve self-support enables a recipient to apply his/her excess income or resources toward occupational goal. Thus, the recipient is providing for the purchase of the plan's objective. Supplemental Security Income does not directly provide funds for the purchase of this objective.

4. A plan to achieve self-support is designed to aid blind and disabled individuals in reducing or eliminating dependency on SSI and related services. A person who can already maintain self-support is not eligible for this exclusion as they have already achieved the objective of a plan. Yet it is recognized that severely impaired persons have exceptional needs and may use this exclusion to upgrade employment.

In closing, it should be emphasized that this exclusion exists to encourage an attempt to become self-supporting. A legitimate plan to achieve this objective should have no difficulty with SSA or DR approval except for procedural problems. Furthermore, even where severe impairments make the feasibility of success questionable, each individual has a right to make the attempt. If problems occur while implementing a plan to achieve self-support, consult the SSA Claims Manual 12260 through 12470.

DEVELOPING ADVOCACY RESOURCES
by Greg Sanders

With disabled movements growing, more and more community organizations are developing advocacy services. This article will help in obtaining the regulatory basis of the SSI programs. Access to the regulatory provisions of the Supplemental Security Income (SSI) system programs is a fundamental aspect of effective advocacy services. Of course, a community service agency will want to expand beyond these programs into other areas such as Retirement Survivor's Disability Insurance (RSDI), Railroad Retirement Benefits, Veteran's Administration, etc. Nonetheless, the SSI related programs are a rational point to begin planned growth.

Background

Prior to January 1974, public assistance for the Aged, Blind and Disabled was established individually by the state governments with substantial federal funding participation. The implementation of SSI on January 1, 1974, federalized assistance as Congress established a minimum monthly benefit level for all needy aged, blind or disabled Americans. This grant is the Supplemental Security Income (SSI) payment and is entirely federal money. To account for cost-of-living variation among the individual states, Congress provided for mandatory and optional supplementation of the federal benefit level with state funds. Mandatory supplementation was enforced to assure that no recipient received less from the new system than they did from the state programs in December, 1973. Optional supplementation simply encouraged states to provide additional assistance. In short, SSI is entirely federal funds, established and regulated by the federal government. A state supplemental payment (SSP) is entirely state funds, established and regulated by the state government. States which provided a supplemental payment could administer the distribution of this payment themselves, or contract with the Social Security Administration (SSA) to administer the state payment. California elected to contract with SSA. Therefore, California recipients receive one check equalling the combined amount of the SSI level and the SSP level. This SSI/SSP check clearly prints "State Payment Included."

Supplemental security income (SSI)

The federal statute which relates to the SSI program is Title XVI of the Social Security Act. The regulations governing SSI are Part 416 of Title 20 of the Code of Federal Regulations. The best source of information on SSI is the Social Security Administration's Claims Manual. The Claims Manual (CM) does not have the force of law, but accurately represents the law and offers substantial explanations and examples. Most aspects of SSI are covered in Parts 12 and 13 of the CM but some aspects duplicate the RSDI program and are discussed in other areas of the CM. Also, the SSA contracts with state agencies to make determinations in disability claims. For this purpose, there is the Disability Insurance State Manual (DISM), which contains instructions from the SSA to the state agencies.

Parts 12 and 13 of the CM and the DISM are available to community service agencies from: The National Senior Citizen Law Center, 1709 West 8th Street, Los Angeles, Calif. 90017. The cost is $20 for the basic material and updating transmittals. Information on SSI which is not in Parts 12 or 13 can be studied at your local SSA office.

State supplementation

California offers significant services beyond the federal SSI benefit. These services involve three major aspects: (1) a state supplemental payment increasing the SSI/SSP monthly maintenance check; (2) a Special Circumstance Payment program offering assistance in certain situations which jeopardize the health and safety of recipients; and (3) a Homemaker and Chore service program offering in-home supportive service necessary to enable aged, blind and disabled persons to remain in their own homes—out of institutions.

State supplemental program

The regulations governing the supplemental payment and the Special Circumstance Payments are presented in the Eligibility Assistance Standards (EAS). The EAS compose part of the Manual on Policies and Procedures (MPP). The State Supplemental Program is presented in Division 46 of the MPP. The EAS also covers the Aid to Potentially Self-Supporting Blind (APSB) program and the Aid to Families with Dependent Children (AFDC) program. To obtain the EAS, write to the Department of Benefit Payments, Publications, 714 "P" Street, Sacramento, Calif. 95814. Request the Eligibility and Assistance Standards, and ask to be placed on the mailing list for updating DBP (Dept. of Benefit Payments) manual letters. Presently, this material is free and delivery is prompt.

Homemaker and chore services

Title XX of the Social Security Act provides federal funding participation to State programs which accomplish certain social service goals. To prevent institutionalization of aged, blind and disabled individuals, California provides In-Home Supportive Service (IHSS) through the Homemaker/Chore (H/C) program. Briefly, Homemaker service provides in-home support when supervision by the provider of service is necessary. Generally, the provider is employed by a private Homemaker agency or a County agency. Chore service provides in-home support for recipients who are capable of administering their own affairs. Chore service may be provided through a direct payment to the recipient who will employ the provider of service; or, the County may employ and pay the provider who is otherwise under the supervision of the recipient. The regulations governing Homemaker and Chore services are in Social Service Standards. These standards comprise Divisions 30 and 31 of the Manual of Policies and Procedures. To obtain this material write to the Department of Health, 744 P Street, Sacramento, Calif. 95814. Request the Social Service Standards and ask to be placed on the mailing list for updating material. This material is free and may be requested by phone—Department of Health, (916) 445-4171.

Medi-Cal

Medicaid is a federal medical coverage program for financially needy Americans. It is established by Title XIX of the Social Security Act. Medi-Cal is California's Medicaid program. Thus, in accordance with federal Medicaid regulations, California established the Medi-Cal program which involves substantial federal funding participation. The entire Medi-Cal program is presented in Title 22 of the California Administrative Code. Recent legislation (Summer, 1976) has substantially changed the Medi-Cal program. The new regulations are presently available in most public libraries and all County Welfare Departments. Title 22 is available from the Department of Health, but the cost is $68.00 plus $8.00 for the annual subscription to updating material. Eventually, the Department of Health may offer key parts of Title 22 to community organizations at a reduced price. Also, a basic layperson's guide to Medi-Cal is available from the State Office on Aging, 455 Capitol Mall, Room 500, Sacramento, Calif. 95814. Request "An Advocate's Basic Guide to Medi-Cal—The California Medical Assistance Program." The guide is free.

Training Material

There are two basic guides on the SSI system developed for laypersons. It may be useful to obtain both manuals.

1. *The Supplemental Security Income System for California's Aged, Blind and Disabled: A Training and Reference Manual* is one of the most readable and useful guides. In addition to SSI, the manual discusses services in California. It is available from:

Assembly Publications
Box 90
State Capitol
Sacramento, Calif. 95814
The cost is $3.30.

2. *The Supplemental Security Income Advocate's Handbook* is a similar manual but offers a national perspective and does not address any particular state. It is available from:

Center on Social Welfare and Public Law
25 West 43rd
New York, New York 10036
The cost is $3.50.

Also, CIL has written discussions on specific issues. If you need information on a specific subject, contact CIL c/o Advocacy Unit. We will provide what material we have, or suggest other reference sources. There may be a small charge for reproduction.

The impact of child-rearing practices on the future of the individual is, without question, enormous. There is no set of plans or blueprint—no universal rules—that can be followed to obtain a finished product of ideal proportions. The imposition of a disability sets into motion a series of decisions and consequences for which there are, again, no specified game plans. The first of the next two articles describes what the author believes to be the primary factor in the development of the child with a physical disability: a lack of a positive self-image, not the disability itself. The second article, by an adult with cerebral palsy, is a reflection on growing up, including the author's confrontation with the reality of who he is in relation to where he has been and his encounters with the outside world that he has had to manage.

RAISING THE DISABLED CHILD
by Peter Leech

Ever since I contracted polio 18 years ago, and especially since I began to practice clinical social work 11 years ago, I've been trying to understand the emotional impact and varied response to disabling illness or injury.

The quality of the response seems to bear no relationship to the magnitude of the injury or disability. Therefore, I have come to believe that the physical damage, however devastating, is really of secondary importance as a disabling factor. Of primary importance is, I believe, the degree to which the individual's self-image is shattered and fails to redevelop as a positive force in the individual's life. In the case of persons disabled from birth or infancy I believe the primary disabling factor to be the failure to develop a positive self-image. I want to discuss some of the factors which I think interfere with the disabled child's development. . . .

Let me hypothesize a bit about the ways in which persons, disabled from birth or infancy, are affected with respect to their development of a positive self-image. I want to point out that when I refer to disability or disabled children, I am speaking of physically exceptional children—those whose injuries or illnesses, whether prenatal, or developed after birth, caused some kind of physical exceptionality—blindness, deafness, paralysis, orthopedic difficulties.

Their caretakers—the persons the child depends on for nurture, love, guidance, protection, etc.—are able-bodied, whether parents, or staff of their institution, or teachers in their school for handicapped children. This may make sense as a practical matter, but provides no person with whom to identify in the process of developing a positive sense of physical self. While physical capability is being applauded all around, the child with a physical disability is neither achieving, nor able to observe physically disabled adults accomplish their living tasks. The result is that positive role-models relating to the physically exceptional body image are absent for the most part from the child's experience.

Overprotection

The tendency for the child's caretakers to "protect the child from further hurt" is a process which often leads to overprotection. The basis for the overprotective approach is undoubtedly as varied as the children, parents, and other caretakers involved, and will be discussed in another paper. The point is that overprotectiveness limits the outer range of the child's experience of what is possible. Of course each child's outer limit will be unique. But rather than allow each child to experience his/her limit, the caretaker chooses, and too often does so in relation to the difference he perceives between the physically exceptional child and an able-bodied child. The statement received by the child in this interaction is something like "You can't do these things because you're physically disabled." And because the source of these statements is the caretaker, they are trusted and believed.

Another factor which inhibits the disabled child's development of a positive self-image is the sense of "not belonging" and isolation which flows out of not being "like" able-bodied people. The caretakers communicate that only that which approaches the cultural norm is acceptable: those activities which are directed toward what is "normal" are encouraged, and those which deviate from normal are discouraged or disallowed.

Independence

It is not important here whether such attitudes originate in the wish that the child not be disabled, or in a lack of vision on the part of the caretakers. What is important is that the isolation which results interferes with disabled childrens' appreciation of their own accomplishments for their own sake. Rather than applaud the child's natural efforts to get around or communicate in whatever manner works best, the child is encouraged to "walk" or "talk." This approach often goes so far as to withhold assistive devices or techniques with the argument that the child will become "too dependent" on them. To withhold a wheelchair to encourage walking, or sign language to encourage talking is to foster dependence on the caretakers for ambulation and interpretation.

Adaptive heritage

I don't believe that people naturally develop a dependent lifestyle; our most distant ancestors were able to survive in primitive circumstances beyond our comprehension. They experimented with assistive devices and techniques, i.e. tools, retaining those that increased their abilities, rejecting those that did not. No one went before, making the selections to prevent their becoming "too dependent." Our children, physically exceptional or not, retain that adaptive heritage, and lose it only through acculturation. We have the technology to help our disabled children to survive; we might exercise the wisdom to allow them to learn to employ on their own behalf whatever further resources are available to assist their growth and independence.

The result, however, of the absence of models, overprotection and isolation is that, too often, persons disabled from infancy reach adulthood with the same attitudes toward themselves as those developed by adults who experience a disabling illness or injury. That is, they feel as though they are—and thus believe they must truly be—invalid, dependent, asexual, ineffective, noncontributory human beings. A different result is accomplished when the disabled child is taught and believes that he is fully a member of the human community.

ON GROWING UP TIGHT
by Michael B. Williams

I've always been a fan of Mary Shelley's Frankenstein's monster. To most people this minor footnote to English literature is just a tale concocted to entertain friends on a winter's eve. To me, however, Mary's brainchild provides a striking metaphor for growing up with cerebral palsy.

Up until a few years ago I considered myself a monster. I walked like a monster, lurching my way along the street, my body performing a strange visual symphony of contractions. When I attempted to speak, I sounded like a monster. All sorts of strange sounds came bubbling out of my mouth. Many people were uncomfortable at the sight of me. They either turned their heads away in fear and embarrassment or gawked in naked curiosity. I was truly a monster.

I have since discovered I'm not the monster I thought. It just lived inside of me, spawned from the culture of narrow social attitudes towards anyone who may be different and nurtured by my own sense of self-isolation.

When you grow up with cerebral palsy, chances are you grow up isolated—first in a padded cell of parental protectiveness, then in special schools that have been so thoughtfully provided for you by the state, and finally, and most completely, by your own fears.

I spent most of my childhood in the company of adults. I spent endless hours on the floor of my parents' living room listening to sterile conversations about new hats, dresses and coats from the ladies, and heated diatribes about That Man in the White House—FDR—from the men.

When I was surfeited by this boredom, I switched on the radio—yes, dear reader, I'm old enough to remember this ancient form of entertainment—and took solace in the troubles of such people as Helen Trent, Pepper Young, and Mary Noble, backstage wife.

Peer group pressure played little part in my development. When I was subjected to it, I was usually snatched from it as if from a flame. Once, when I was about four, I was playing in a sandbox with a friend. I was hogging the shovel and my friend decided to give me an object lesson in the art of sharing. He snatched the shovel from my hand and hit me over the head with it, cutting me rather badly.

From that point on my mother took over management of my alter ego. Whenever I entered a new area of experience, my mother always would pave the way for me. I always let her. After all, it was so much easier than doing it myself. I couldn't talk, she was very articulate. She always said the things I would say.

This had a subtle but profound effect on my personality. When you have someone representing you at the bargaining table of life, all you have to do is sit back and reap the benefits. As a result, I didn't develop my sense of anger and outrage until recently. All I had to do was sit there and be Mr. Nice Guy while my mother took care of the flack coming down on me.

I realize I haven't mentioned my father in all this. I'm still trying to figure out where he fit into the scheme of things. He was a very shadowy figure in my life. He had very skilled hands that could fashion any piece of wood or metal into a thing of beauty. My hands were twisted and could barely perform a simple task of buttoning a button. I was an English major. My father read few books during his lifetime. He made his living designing weapon systems. I was a pacifist. We had little to discuss with each other.

My father died in 1966, six months after my mother. I've thought about my father a lot these past eight years. He must have been a very lonely and unhappy man. I drew much of the attention and love he rightfully deserved. My parents' marriage was over long before they died. I know this not from what they said or did, but from what they did not do and did not say. I guess both of them lacked the courage to call it quits and waited for Death to pull the last strands of a tenuous relationship apart.

Their death had a devastating effect on me. The monster was now alone in the world. He had a mouthpiece no longer. He was on his own.

Well, I spent the first six months of my "independence" holed up in a five room house which I now owned, listening to rock music and dancing a furious and concerted dance until I fell over in a heap. It wasn't a very creative period. I tried to spice up my ennui via a lukewarm suicide attempt, complete with music by Leonard Cohen on the stereo. All I succeeded in doing was to prove poor intentions make poor art.

I decided to move to Hollywood, mainly because I had friends there and because I was living in Altadena, a town that's as exciting as a broken kiddy car.

These first few years on my own were extremely rough. I was in a peer group situation for the first time in my life, coming to terms with my disability, having to cope with my anger and thinking things I'd never thought about before, like sex.

About my anger I can only say I repressed it to the extreme. Whenever a point of contention arose between me and the people I was living with, I'd always concede it to them out of fear. I was afraid if I became the least bit testy, I would soon have no friends. After all, who likes an angry monster?

By far the most difficult problem I've had to face has been the matter of sex. When most of the people are having successful love relationships, it is extremely painful to go to bed every night alone. Whenever a potential relationship with a woman doesn't blossom, I'm tempted to fall back on the lame excuse (pun intended) of nobody loves a monster, especially one who talks funny, moves with the grace of a wounded elephant and who drools on occasion. But then I realize that I'm just suffering the consequences of all those years I spent isolated from society. It's just the interest that's accrued from growing up tight.

Persons with physical disabilities are sexual persons. They can have active sex lives and have sexual needs the same as persons without disabilities. Among the problems associated with disability, sexual functioning has only recently been given much attention. Other levels of physical functioning, such as walking and self-care abilities, have been part of the concern of the professional community for years. When sex reared its ugly head, however, the topic was ignored, poorly discussed, or rejected as unnecessary. The following article reveals some of the frustrations and needs for understanding and education that a person with a disability may have with regard to sexual functioning and sexuality.

GETTING THERE IS HALF THE FUN—THE SEXUALLY ACTIVE QUAD
by Scott Luebking

I was nineteen when I broke my neck and entered quad-dom. I had been very sexually active. (Being young, I didn't need much rest.)

After my accident, I had questions about my sexual capacity. It became obvious that I wouldn't have to worry about getting erections. But I kept getting it up at the strangest times, like in the middle of watching Sesame Street. I was concerned. Had I developed a fetish for Big Bird?

So I knew about my erections. But what about the rest of my sexual functions? At the rehabilitation center the doctors told me about skin care. The physical therapists explained to me about range of motion. The occupational therapists showed me how to eat. But as for sex . . . Well, I guess they didn't think that was an "Activity for Daily Living."

After six months, on a Saturday, I left Rehab and moved directly into a dorm at my old college. Two days later I started spring quarter carrying a full course load. I also started doing work with my usual campus organizations.

It was a hard quarter. Wheelchair breakdowns, catheter problems, trying to handle old situations with a new body.

The quarter was finally over. I finished by making the Dean's list and a suicide attempt.

That summer I got into a couple of situations which could have been sexual, but avoided that aspect. I was scared. I didn't know what would happen. And then I decided I had to know.

I made an appointment with my physiatrist, a doctor of physiotherapy. Went down to the office. Closed the door. Looked at her grey hair and veined hands. Thought of my grandmother. And promptly asked her about . . . my ingrown toenail.

Still sexually ignorant, I returned to school that fall.

I got pretty good at avoiding sexual situations. At one party, this girl began to make all sorts of advances. She kept attacking and I realized that she was going to sit on my lap. Just as she was in midflight, I noted to her an interesting, but, I'm afraid, fictitious point. I claimed that my legbag was full and that if she sat on my lap, we'd have Lake Luebking all over the floor—and her.

She was kind of grossed out and left me alone for the rest of the night.

The following February, an interesting thing happened. I got laid. It was the first time since my accident. Both of us were only partially satisfied.

But in a way it was great. Not because of what had happened, but because it had happened at all. It got in touch with the parts of my body below my chest, which I had rejected after my accident. I was beginning to be sexual again—a member of the human race.

But I hadn't ejaculated. I hadn't had an orgasm. And I wasn't sure it was possible. May be I needed to be stimulated more or in some particular way. I just didn't know.

During subsequent sexual encounters, I became more proficient at satisfying my partners. And since I was being successful, I kept doing it. But my partners didn't know how to satisfy me and I couldn't help them.

That summer I went to my new physiatrist. He asked me about my skin, my bladder, and my sex life. Skin and bladder were fine. But my sex life . . . Still, two out of three isn't bad.

So we rapped about it. My suspicions about being incapable of ejaculation were confirmed. And he pretty much said that the only pleasure I'd get would be from satisfying my partner.

But damn it! I was tired of playing Santa Claus. I wanted something in return, not just gold stars for performance. Even though I couldn't feel pain and temperature, I could still sense pressure. And something should be able to be done with that!

But next year, my final year in college, was great. I had become something of a success story. Studied acting. Got accepted into the computer science doctorate program at Berkeley. Finally graduated with a Phi Beta Kappa key.

Sexually, the year had been a bust.

When I got to Berkeley, things began to change. Here, I encountered someone who was less genitally oriented and more into a whole-body experience. I found parts of my body that I hadn't known to be so sensitive. My feet and neck are extremely so. And I found I could really get turned on.

But I was still unsure of myself. So I sought help. Finally tracked down Sue Knight and Bob Geiger at the Human Sexuality Program at the University of California Medical Center. I went to see them and all of us were surprised. They, because of how together I was sexually, having been a quad only three years. I, because of how surprised they were.

Through their reactions I gained a lot of confidence in where I was at sexually and in being on the right track of a whole-body experience.

But there was still some doubt. It was of the type that words could not drive away. It had to be dispelled by successful experience. And so for the next five months, I was incredibly promiscuous. And I mean promiscuous, like sometimes five different partners in one week. But it worked. My worries about my sexuality were replaced by ones concerning treatment of scabbies.

With all these experiences, I was able to explore a lot of different things and come up with some interesting ideas. I'd like to pass on some of these observations.

One thing I got in touch with is that often the disabled person has to take care of the able-bodied. I know this sounds strange, but the "crip" has to do this if he wants to get any place, and I found that the means is through communication.

What do I mean by "take care of"? Well, a lot of able-bodied people have had some strange notions put into their heads. They may feel afraid of looking at a disabled person for fear of being thought of as staring. Or even if full of questions, they may completely avoid talking about the disability because they don't want to embarrass the disabled person. In this case, I take care of the able-bodied by somehow working into the conversation that I had a diving accident and am a quadriplegic as a result. In this way I try to tell them that it's all right to ask me about my disability and that I won't be embarrassed by their questions. And so, by taking care of the able-bodied person, I also take care of myself.

Here are some other examples of how I take care of an able-bodied person through communication. If I'm interested in a person sexually, I am sure to convey the fact that I am very much sexual in spite of being disabled. (Many able-bodied people assume that I and other disabled are not sexual.) I explain to my partner how to transfer me into bed, and how to undress me. I'm also careful to reassure that I'm not fragile and won't break if dropped. (And making it on the floor can be interesting anyway.) I explain about my physiology, what I can do in bed, and what really turns me on. Again, how can I assume that the person will know all this?

On the other hand, this principle also applies to me. How do I know what turns my partner on? And so, if I haven't been told, I take the initiative and ask. I feel that this, plus getting into a more whole-body orientation, has made me a much better lover than I was before my accident.

Here's another way I take care of an able-bodied person. I am sure to tell the person that it's all right to say "no" to me. Many able-bodied people feel that if asked by a disabled person to have sex with him, they should agree. After all, the poor guy is crippled.

But I don't want or need sympathetic sex. I like friendly sex. And so I'm careful to give people permission to say "no" when I ask to have sex with them or in fact, do almost anything for me. It helps avoid guilt, resentment, and anger, enemies of any close relationship.

Another concept some doctors over at the Human Sexuality Program of the University of California Medical Center have come up with, is that of a non-genitally based orgasm in men. There's a fair amount of evidence to support this idea.

Masters and Johnson did research concerning breast stimulation in women. They discovered an interesting thing about some of their subjects. These women were having orgasms when just their breasts were fondled and their genitals not even touched. If women can get off with nongenital stimulation, why not men? Is their physiology that different? I think not.

Another piece of evidence is that some quads with completely transected spinal cords have reported having orgasms in their dreams. Their spinal cords do not miraculously repair during the night. Yet, they are experiencing orgasms. This leads one to suspect that the most sexual organ in a person's body is not between their legs, but between their ears.

In my experience with sex I have found that I can get extremely turned on by stimulation to non-genital areas. My neck is extremely sensitive. Sometimes it's hard to let anyone even touch it because of such powerful sensations. And I feel that with enough work, I'll eventually have orgasms just by non-genital stimulation.

But will that be a real orgasm? I had orgasms before my accident and I know what they're like. If I think that I am experiencing an orgasm, can anyone deny that that's what I am feeling? And so what if ejaculation doesn't occur? Ejaculation is a physiological response. Orgasm is psychological.

Now comes the question of just how important is having an orgasm. I compare sex to taking a trip to Colorado. You can go to Colorado and really enjoy yourself there. But you can also enjoy the scenes on the way to and back. And what if you don't reach your destination? You can still have a lot of fun just travelling and exploring various routes.

It is often said that truth is stranger than fiction. One reason for this much repeated expression may be that truth includes everything that is present and real, whereas fiction can, at the drop of a pen, delete or change anything that is unappealing. How successful would "Ironside" have been if the truth were known?

IRONSIDE: STRANGER IN A STRANGE LAND
by Phil Draper

Disabled people know that there are many real and important everyday problems that are never mentioned or dealt with on *Ironside*. Here is a story about Ironside that should make him a little more real life.

Time: Yesterday, today, and tomorrow.

Mark, the young black man who is Ironside's attendant, has just arrived. He has been partying all night and looks and feels it. Sullen and hungover, his thoughts run on about the day's work ahead.

"Hmmph . . . Late as usual!" grumbles Ironside. All the same, he's thankful for the opportunity to lie in bed a few extra minutes.

The confrontation is typical. Mark, knowing that his boss is faking sleep, grabs the covers and throws them back. "Time to get up, Chief."

Ironside screams like a man who has just been thrown into an icy river. "How many times have I told you not to do that, especially when I'm sleeping, and besides, it's colder'n . . ."

Mark winces at the shrill sound emoting from the huge object lying in bed.

"Look man, don't be coming down on me! It's always too hot in here any-way."

Ironside grabs the blankets and pulls them up around his head, eyes and nose barely exposed. "While I'm trying to get warm, go and put my irrigation utensils on to boil. Also, my urine bag needs to be cleaned out."

Mark leaves the room grumbling.

Meanwhile, Ironside is contemplating whether or not to chance taking his suppository this morning. "If past bowel-care mornings are any indication," he ponders, "it's best not to 'cause I'm tired of accidents and I'll bet Mark is too."

Mark returns with a glove on one hand and silver bullet (suppository) in the other. "Say man, you warm now. We better start taking care of business. You know we got to meet with Mrs. Fredonia about the cat burglar."

"I know all about what I gotta do. I was thinking of doing the silver bullet trip this evening, but since you've got everything ready, I might as well do it now and get it over with, I hope."

"Say, you got a red spot on your tailbone."

"Oh yeah! Is it real red or just red?"

"Well, it ain't too bad."

"I'm sure glad it's Friday so I can stay off it this weekend."

Four hours later, somewhere in hilly San Francisco, a nightmare for anyone in a wheelchair to live, Mark is pushing Ironside to his appointment with Mrs. Fredonia. "I sure would appreciate it if the Chief would lose some weight," he complains to himself.

Mark and Ironside approach the fashionable apartment building where Mrs. Fredonia lives and immediately they notice the 7 steps at its entrance. Ironside, still in a bad mood from the morning, grumbles, "I'm getting tired of being pulled up stairs, and if it's not stairs it's curbs."

Mark: "Yeah, well I'm getting tired too." Mark decides to ask the first person who comes along to help him get Ironside up the stairs.

Later we find Ironside and Mark going over the case with Mrs. Fredonia, the victim of a burglary. "I had just gotten back to bed after feeding Hesperus. You know she's been so picky lately about her food. We had been eating a lot of caviar, but my doctor tells me that eggs are bad for me—high blood pressure you know. So tonight we had sturgeon in a very nice white wine sauce with mushrooms. You don't think that's too commonplace for Hesperus, do you? She seemed to like it. Poor Hesperus! You will find her, won't you?"

"Let's get back to the burglary, Mrs. Fredonia. After feeding your cat, you went back to bed to finish *Stranger in a Strange Land* when you heard a strange sound coming from the bathroom. Would you tell us more about . . . uh . . . the . . . uh . . . mmmm . . . strange. . . uh . . . strange . . .

Suddenly without warning there comes a strange sound that is unfamiliar to most but not to a select few. Ironside, thinking back to the morning, regrets not having postponed the silver bullet trip till the evening. With reddened face, he says, in a disgusted voice, "We'll have to continue this questioning next week. Let's go Mark."

As they approach the elevator, Mark says, "Uh, Chief, if you don't mind, while you take the elevator, I think I'll take the stairs."

SUMMARY

This chapter has explored the functioning and characteristics of adults who are disabled. The various follow-up studies of special education graduates have not shown high levels of successful adult independent living or participation in society. However, we are in a new era, and the adult with a physical disability is no longer willing to accept the societal role of recipient of sympathy, aid, and inadequate education.

The lives of many adults with disabilities are being changed by the opportunities that are being provided by work training and programs in colleges and universities for students with disabilities. Employment for those with disabilities have in the past been most often thought of in terms of agency services such as those provided by Goodwill Industries. Although this organization and others like it have provided a needed training ground and employment opportunity through their sheltered workshops, they foster the notion that this is where the adult with a disability can best function in the world of work. There are few generalizations that could be more damaging to the concept that properly trained or educated persons with disabilities can work and be competitive in the open marketplace.

Special student centers on college and university campuses are providing a variety of services to students with special needs. These services—special parking areas; advanced registration times; special counseling centers; advocacy for student rights; elimination of architectural, housing, and social barriers; and tutorial services—are attracting more students with physical disabilities to higher education than ever before. These students, who become qualified graduates, are now demanding that they be given equal consideration for jobs. They are no longer a quiet minority. This acknowledgment of rights and a recognition of the necessity for social need fulfillment are making the adult with a disability a visible and viable member of society.

REFERENCES

Bachmann, W. H. *Influence of selected variables upon economic adaptation of orthopedically handicapped and other health impaired.* Unpublished doctoral dissertation, University of the Pacific, 1971.

Berry, D. Finding a good attendant. *The Independent*, 1977, *3*, 24.

Brieland, D. A follow-up study of orthopedically handicapped high school graduates. *Exceptional Children*, 1967, *33*, 555-562.

Draper, P. Ironside: stranger in a strange land. *The Independent*, 1977, *3*, 22.

Klapper, Z. S., and Birch, H. G. The relation of childhood characteristics to outcome in young adults with cerebral palsy. *Developmental Medicine and Child Neurology*, 1966, *8*, 645-656.

Leech, P. Raising the disabled child. *The Independent*, 1977, *3*, 16-17.

Luebking, S. Getting there is half the fun—the sexually active quad. *The Independent*, 1977, *3*, 20-21.

Olshansky, S., and Beach, D. A five year follow-up of physically disabled clients. *Rehabilitation Literature*, 1975, *36*, 251-252; 258.

Park, L. D. Barriers to normality for the handicapped adult in the United States. *Rehabilitation Literature*, 1975, *36*, 108-111.

Sanders, G. Developing advocacy resources. *The Independent*, 1977, *3*, 14-15. (a)

Sanders, G. Mobility in bed. *The Independent*, 1977, *3*, 8. (b)

Sanders, G. Plans to achieve self-support. *The Independent*, 1977, *3*, 9-13. (c)

Stein, K. You *can* fight city hall! *The Independent*, 1977, *3*, 6.

Vogel, H. D. A follow-up study of former student-patients at the crippled children's hospital and school, Sioux Falls, South Dakota. *Rehabilitation Literature*, 1975, *36*, 270-273.

Williams, M. B. On growing up tight. *The Independent*, 1977, *3*, 18-19.

Zukas, H. Why disabled people do not use BART (technically accessible). *The Independent*, 1977, *3*, 7.

9 Trends and implications for the future

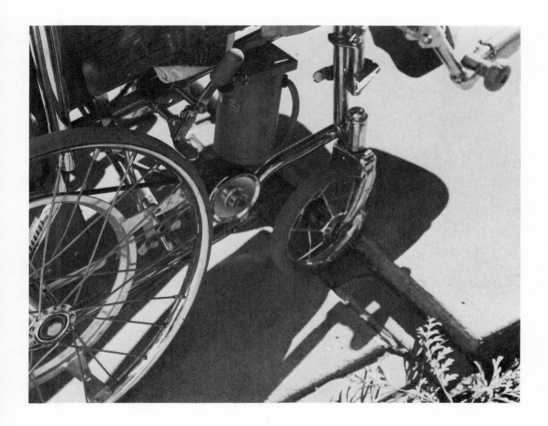

When this book is read, the future at the time of this writing will have become the present or the past for the reader. To look into the future is crystal ball gazing at its worst. And yet, one cannot help but think about what the future will hold— about what the consequences will be of what is now known about physical disability and about what might happen to change the nature of physical disability. If the future is shaped by the past—and it seems likely that it is—and if it is true that there are specific events in history that strongly influence the direction of the future, then the implementation of PL 94-142, the Education for All Handicapped Children Act of 1975, will be a historical milestone.

There will be many interpretations of this law with regard to what its most important features are. These interpretations will be specific to the interests and perspective of the reader and not without value. Four main characteristics of the law are herein identified as having high levels of significance: Who will be educated? Where will they be educated? How will they be educated? *and* What are the procedural safeguards?

WHO WILL BE EDUCATED?

The answer to *who* will be educated is quite clear: *all* handicapped children, as identified in the title of the law. According to the various sections of this law, children between the ages of 3 and 21 shall be provided a free appropriate public education no later than September 1, 1980. Within this age span, certain exceptions may be made for children between 3 and 5 years of age and between 18 and 21 years of age when "such requirements would be inconsistent with a state law or practice, or the order of any court, respecting public education within such age groups in the State" (PL 94-142, Section 162).

In addition to the age range of children to be served as stated in the law, the significant wording with regard to *all* handicapped children is in the phrase stating that children will be identified and served regardless of the severity of their handicap.

Why are these statements part of the law? The reason seems to be because of the overwhelming number of children who have not been identified as needing special education services and/or who have not been provided for. According to the law itself, over 4 million handicapped children have not received an appropriate education for full equality of opportunity, and 1 million handicapped children have been excluded entirely from public education. Many of these children have gone unidentified; in many instances, there have not been programs available for these children even if they were known to the school system. With the requirement that all children be identified and served regardless of the severity of handicap, a large number of children who are severely retarded or multihandicapped will now be served. Thompson (1976) has provided figures showing that these two groups alone account for nearly one half million children. The presence of disabilities in these children is a given, and no longer will it be sufficient for the teacher of children with physical disabilities to be trained to be responsible educationally just for those children described in Chapter 1. Although there will be children with physical disabilities in the range of severity described throughout this book, teachers will need to be increasingly aware of the potential for placement of children in their classroom who may be severely involved with multiple disabilities—or of the potential for having a class totally composed of such children. This awareness will have to go beyond a nodding acceptance of the presence of these children; it will have to take the form of additional training and expectation for teaching this part of the population referred to as *all* handicapped children.

The impact of this legislation lies in the acknowledgement that all children have the right to be taught, that there are appropriate levels of education that can be presented, that there are techniques and equipment available for utilization, and the need, above all, that these children are a part of us all. What now challenges society is the need to make provisions within its social framework for a space for these children once they have been provided the opportunity to develop to their maximum. If this is not done, then what has been accomplished is little more than what is accomplished when one blows air into a paper bag.

WHERE WILL THEY BE EDUCATED?

The question of *where* they will be educated might be expanded to include *with whom* they will be educated.

> . . . to the maximum extent appropriate, handicapped children including children in public or private institutions or other care facilities . . . [will be] educated with children who are not handicapped, and special classes, separate schooling, or other removal of handicapped children from the regular educational environment . . . [will occur] only when the nature or severity of the handicap is such that education in regular classes with the use of supplementary aids and services cannot be achieved satisfactorily, . . . (PL 94-142, Section 612)

This requirement, referred to as the *least restrictive environment,* provides that, to the extent possible, handicapped children will no longer be apart from society by educational fiat but will be a part of society. The special class and school will no longer be the exclusive learning environment for the child with a disability. And so, a progression is seen from the voluntary integration of children with physical disabilities into classes of nondisabled children, to the era of mainstreaming fostered by Dunn's (1968) accusations of inadequate education for children with social needs, to federal mandate for learning in the least restrictive environment.

Children with physical disabilities who are able to function in classes and schools with their nondisabled peers will see benefits from two directions: there will be an opportunity for social interaction with peers throughout their educational careers, and the nondisabled peers will have the same opportunity to learn about their colleagues with disabilities. It is an important part of learning and living to understand that being chosen last to be on a team may be a consequence of disability and will have to be dealt with as part of living with nondisabled peers. As difficult as it may be, there is a need to face this prospect; and this need is denied if the child with a disability is not included in the regular education placement. Placement in a special school with no interaction with others except those with disabilities eliminates the possibility of being selected to participate in an activity with nondisabled classmates—there are no nondisabled classmates in the special school.

It must be realized, however, that there are some circumstances, medical conditions, and individual needs that are best met in a special setting. These needs will not go unmet as a result of this new legislation. Special classes and schools, instruction in the home, and instruction in hospitals and institutions are not denied to those who need them; they will, as a matter of course, be available to children whose needs cannot be achieved satisfactorily in educational placements with nonhandicapped peers.

HOW WILL THEY BE EDUCATED?

Of the several parts of the new law providing education to all handicapped children, the section that relates to the educational program of the child has probably had the most immediate impact on teachers. Known as an "individualized educational program" (IEP), the section from the law defining this term is presented here:

> . . . a written statement for each handicapped child developed in any meeting by a representative of the local educational agency or an intermediate educational unit who shall be qualified to provide, or supervise the provision of, specially designed instruction to meet the unique needs of handicapped children, the teacher, the parents or guardian of such children, and whenever appropriate, such child, which statement shall include (A) a statement of the present levels of educational performance of such child, (B) a statement of annual goals, including short-term instructional objectives, (C) a statement of the specific educational services to be provided to such child, and the extent to which such child will be able to participate in regular educational programs, (D) the projected date for initiation and anticipated duration of such services, and appropriate objective criteria and evaluation procedures and schedules for determining, on at least an annual basis, whether instructional objectives are being achieved. (PL 94-142, Section 4)

That the IEP will be developed in a meeting, rather than in isolation by any single party, is clear, as is the fact that the parents will be included in the process of planning for their child. Also of significance is the individual aspect of the plan—that a plan will be developed for each handicapped child.

Less specific and left to the elaboration of educational agencies are the points concerning (1) what constitutes present levels of educational performance; (2)

what the characteristics are of statements of goals and short-term objectives, particularly as these statements refer to time references and to methods and criteria for measurement; (3) the nature of special education and related services that are to be provided; (4) the participation of the child in regular education; (5) the dates and immediacy of implementation and continuation of the program; and (6) the specifics regarding the timing and criteria for an annual review of the program.

That state and local educational agencies will refine and develop procedures and formats for the preparation and implementation of IEPs is certain.

In addition to requirements of IEP development, safeguards for the evaluation and assessment of children are cited in the law. These safeguards are related to the nondiscriminatory techniques of evaluation for purposes of eliminating cultural and communication disadvantages.

Putting aside these educational practices that are required by law, one should probably give consideration to why these requirements have become "the law of the land." For every specific requirement stated in the law (the requirement of education for *all* children, nondiscriminatory evaluation, parental involvement, and all the others), practices relating to the requirement have been denied or have not been available to these children, their parents, and educators. The denial of rights can no longer be part of the educational and social conditions of persons with disabilities.

WHAT ARE THE PROCEDURAL SAFEGUARDS?

The law has provided for a structure in which the rights made available under the act are now protected through procedural due process. All three parties to the implementation of the law—the child, the parents, and the schools—are involved in the specifics of the due process. As outlined by Abeson and Zettel (1977), the elements of due process include:

1. Written notification before evaluation. In addition, the right to an interpreter/translator if the family's native language is not English (unless it is clearly not feasible to do so).
2. Written notification when initiating or refusing to initiate a change in educational placement.
3. Opportunity to present complaints regarding the identification, evaluation, placement, or the provision of a free appropriate education.
4. Opportunity to obtain an independent educational evaluation of the child.
5. Access to all relevant records.
6. Opportunity for an impartial due process hearing including the right to:
   a. Receive timely and specific notice of the hearing.
   b. Be accompanied and advised by counsel and by individuals with

special knowledge or training with respect to the problems of children with handicaps.

c. Confront, cross-examine, and compel the attendance of witnesses.

d. Present evidence:
   (1) Written or electronic verbatim record of the hearing.
   (2) Written findings of fact and decisions.

7. The right to appeal the findings and decisions of the hearing. (pp. 125-126)*

Why the insistence on due process? A long and involved answer is unnecessary. "School personnel as well as parents can use these procedures to insure that what is required—the appropriate education of the child—is achieved" (Abeson and Zettel, 1977, p. 126).

THE LIBERATED DISABLED: FACT, FICTION, OR FANTASY?

Bills of rights such as those stated in Chapter 1 are statements of what ought to be. There is today a movement away from statements of what ought to be toward what must be. And, like the Bill of Rights of the United States Constitution, these statements of what must be are now taking the form of law. The preceding discussion of PL 94-142 is a statement of what must be. It is fact, not fiction or fantasy of what ought to be.

Another important statement in the form of law that supports the rights of persons with disabilities is found in the Rehabilitation Act of 1973:

> . . . no otherwise qualified handicapped individual . . . shall, solely by reason of his handicap, be excluded from the participation in, be denied the benefits of, or be subjected to discrimination under any program or activity receiving federal financial assistance. (PL 93-112, Section 504)

With the threat of withdrawal of the massive amounts of federal support for industry and for educational and other social institutions where discriminatory practices in employment or in activities and programs are exercised solely on the basis of disability, a level of participation by persons with disabilities in the overall social structure will be enhanced as at no other time in our history. This too is fact, not fiction or fantasy of what ought to be.

Are persons with disabilities liberated? In the sense that there are now statutes enforcing a level of rightful participation in society, the answer may be yes. Groups of persons with disabilities can, and do, exert a political force and cohesiveness. But restrictions remain. Housing is still inadequate in availability for independent living by many persons with physical disabilities. Transportation is likewise inac-

---

*Reprinted from The end of the quiet revolution: the Education for All Handicapped Children Act of 1975 by A. Abeson and J. Zettel, *Exceptional Children*, 1977, *44*, 114-128, by permission of the Council for Exceptional Children; copyright 1977 by the Council for Exceptional Children, 1920 Association Drive, Reston, Va. 22091.

cessible to these persons. Above all, there are the doors to social acceptance that still must be opened beyond the crack now achieved. The dead bolts and chain locks must be removed so that all of our citizens can exercise the freedoms and rights that are available.

Acceptance of one another cannot be mandated or legislated. However, the restrictions that have forbidden access of some individuals to others can be eliminated, so that opportunities for becoming part of something great are available and the choice of participation is extended to all.

SUMMARY

Some of the major components of legislation that have brought the opportunity for equal education to all handicapped children have been reviewed. Although only a portion of PL 94-142 is presented here, it is suggested that the reader secure a copy of the law and study it in its entirety.

As a final suggestion for consideration, the following is offered: Be adventurous in knowing people. Do not seek out persons with disabilities; seek out persons without regard to ability or disability. Broaden your horizons so that you may become and help others become better individuals.

REFERENCES

Abeson, A., and Zettel, J. The end of the quiet revolution: the Education for All Handicapped Children Act of 1975. *Exceptional Children,* 1977, *44,* 114-128.

Dunn, L. M. Special education for the mildly retarded: is much of it justifiable? *Exceptional Children,* 1968, *35,* 5-22.

PL 93-112. *Rehabilitation Act of 1973.*

PL 94-142. *Education for All Handicapped Children Act of 1975.*

Thompson, R. P. The severely handicapped: a new horizon. *Exceptional Children,* 1976, *43,* 141-142.

APPENDIXES

Organizations providing
information and services

Allergy Foundation of America
801 Second Ave.
New York, N.Y. 10017

American Academy of Allergy
225 E. Michigan
Milwaukee, Wis. 53202

American Academy for Cerebral Palsy
1255 New Hampshire Ave. N.W.
Washington, D.C. 20036

American Academy of Pediatrics
1801 Hinman Ave.
Evanston, Ill. 60204

American Academy of Physical Medicine
and Rehabilitation
30 N. Michigan Ave.
Chicago, Ill. 60602

American Association for Clinical
Immunology and Allergy
P.O. Box 912 DTS
Omaha, Neb. 68101

American Association for Health, Physical
Education, and Recreation
1201 16th St. N.W.
Washington, D.C. 20036

American Association on Mental
Deficiency
5201 Connecticut Ave. N.W.
Washington, D.C. 20015

Most of these organizations have journals and
newsletters available to members and to others for
a fee. Requests should be made directly to the
organization.

American Association for Rehabilitation
Therapy
P.O. Box 93
North Little Rock, Ark. 72116

American Association for Respiratory
Therapy
7411 Hines Pl.
Dallas, Tex. 75235

American Association for Study of
Neoplastic Diseases
10607 Miles Ave.
Cleveland, Ohio 44105

American Cancer Society
777 Third Ave.
New York, N.Y. 10017

American Corrective Therapy Association
6622 Spring Hollow
San Antonio, Tex. 78249

American Epilepsy Society
Division of Neurosurgery
University of Texas Medical Branch
Galveston, Tex. 77550

American Health Foundation
1370 Avenue of the Americas
New York, N.Y. 10019

American Heart Association
7320 Greenville Ave.
Dallas, Tex. 75231

American Lung Association
1740 Broadway
New York, N.Y. 10019

American Occupational Therapy
Association
6000 Executive Blvd., Suite 200
Rockville, Md. 20852

American Orthopaedic Association
430 N. Michigan Ave.
Chicago, Ill. 60611

American Orthopsychiatric Association
1775 Broadway
New York, N.Y. 10019

American Orthotic and Prosthetic
Association
14444 N. St. N.W.
Washington, D.C. 20005

American Parkinson Disease Association
147 E. 50th St.
New York, N.Y. 10022

American Physical Therapy Association
1156 15th St. N.W.
Washington, D.C. 20005

American Public Health Association
1015 18th St. N.W.
Washington, D.C. 20036

American Rehabilitation Counseling
Association
1607 New Hampshire Ave. N.W.
Washington, D.C. 20009

American Rheumatism Association
475 Riverside Dr.
New York, N.Y. 10027

American School Health Association
Kent, Ohio 44240

American Thyroid Association
Mayo Clinic
Rochester, Minn. 55901

American Urological Association
1120 N. Charles St.
Baltimore, Md. 21201

Architectural Barriers Committee
National Association of the Physically
Handicapped
6473 Grandville
Detroit, Mich. 48228

Arthritis Foundation
475 Riverside Dr., Rm. 240
New York, N.Y. 10027

Association for the Care of Children
in Hospitals
P.O. Box H
Union, W.Va. 24983

Center for Independent Living, Inc.
2539 Telegraph Ave.
Berkeley, Calif. 94704

Children's Asthma Research Institute and
Hospital
AKA National Asthma Center
1999 Julian St.
Denver, Colo. 80204

Children's Blood Foundation
342 Madison Ave.
New York, N.Y. 10017

Council for Exceptional Children
1920 Association Dr.
Reston, Va. 22091

Cystic Fibrosis Foundation
3379 Peachtree Rd. N.E.
Atlanta, Ga. 30326

Epilepsy Foundation of America
1828 L St. N.W., Suite 406
Washington, D.C. 20036

Foundation for Child Development
345 E. 46th St.
New York, N.Y. 10017

Goodwill Industries of America
9200 Wisconsin Ave.
Washington, D.C. 20014

Heart and Lung Foundation
1025 Fifth Ave.
New York, N.Y. 10028

Hemophilia Research
60 E. 42nd St.
New York, N.Y. 10017

Indoor Sports Club
1145 Highland St.
Napoleon, Ohio 43545

International Society for Rehabilitation of
the Disabled
122 E. 23rd St.
New York, N.Y. 10010

Juvenile Diabetes Foundation
23 E. 26th St.
New York, N.Y. 10010

Leukemia Society of America
211 E. 43rd St.
New York, N.Y. 10017

Muscular Dystrophy Associations
810 Seventh Ave.
New York, N.Y. 10019

Myasthenia Gravis Foundation
230 Park Ave.
New York, N.Y. 10017

National Amputation Foundation
12-45 150th St.
Whitestone, N.Y. 11357

National Association of the Physically
Handicapped
76 Elm St.
London, Ohio 43140

National Association of Private Schools for
Exceptional Children
7700 Miller Rd.
Miami, Fla. 33155

National Association for Retarded Citizens
2709 Avenue E E.
Arlington, Tex. 76011

National Association of State Directors of
Special Education
1510 H St. N.W., Suite 301C
Washington, D.C. 20005

National Ataxia Foundation
4225 Golden Valley Rd.
Minneapolis, Minn. 55422

National Cancer Foundation
1 Park Ave.
New York, N.Y. 10016

National Center on Educational Media and
Materials for the Handicapped
Ohio State University
Columbus, Ohio 43210

National Congress of Organizations of the
Physically Handicapped
7611 Oakland Ave.
Minneapolis, Minn. 55423

National Easter Seal Society for Crippled
Children and Adults
2023 W. Ogden Ave.
Chicago, Ill. 60612

National Foundation—March of Dimes
P.O. Box 2000
White Plains, N.Y. 10602

National Genetics Foundation
9 W. 57th St.
New York, N.Y. 10019

National Heart and Lung Institute
National Institutes of Health
9600 Rockville Pike, Bldg. 31, Rm. 5A52
Bethesda, Md. 20014

National Hemophilia Foundation
25 W. 39th St.
New York, N.Y. 10018

National Institute of Arthritis, Metabolism,
and Digestive Diseases
National Institutes of Health
Bethesda, Md. 20014

National Kidney Foundation
116 E. 27th St.
New York, N.Y. 10016

National Multiple Sclerosis Society
257 Park Ave. S.
New York, N.Y. 10010

National Paraplegia Foundation
333 N. Michigan Ave.
Chicago, Ill. 60601

National Parkinson Foundation
1501 N.W. Ninth Ave.
Miami, Fla. 33136

National Rehabilitation Association
1522 K St. N.W.
Washington, D.C. 20005

National Sudden Infant Death Syndrome
  Foundation
310 S. Michigan Ave.
Chicago, Ill. 60604

National Tay-Sachs and Allied Diseases
  Association
122 E. 42nd St.
New York, N.Y. 10017

National Therapeutic Recreation Society
c/o National Recreation and Park
  Association
1601 N. Kent St.
Arlington, Va. 22209

National Wheelchair Athletic Association
40-24 62nd St.
Woodside, N.Y. 11377

National Wheelchair Basketball
  Association
110 Seaton Bldg.
University of Kentucky
Lexington, Ky. 40506

Parkinson's Disease Foundation
640 W. 168th St.
New York, N.Y. 10032

Sickle Cell Disease Foundation of Greater
  New York
144 W. 125th St.
New York, N.Y. 10027

Society for the Rehabilitation for the Facially
  Disfigured
550 First Ave.
New York, N.Y. 10016

United Cerebral Palsy Association
66 E. 34th St.
New York, N.Y. 10016

B Books "more readable" than textbooks

The books included in this appendix are not textbooks and may have considerably more appeal than many of the tomes of the professional literature. A sizable library of fiction has portrayed those with disabilities in negative or villainous or, at least, in highly sympathetic roles—Captain Hook of *Peter Pan,* Long John Silver of *Treasure Island,* Quasimodo of *The Hunchback of Notre Dame,* Lord Chatterly of *Lady Chatterly's Lover,* and, of course, Tiny Tim of *A Christmas Carol* are examples. The books listed here, however, written by and about persons with physical disabilities, are, in most instances, accurate in clinical detail and highly responsive to the social and personal aspects of disability. They have been written for children and adults and represent only a small proportion of fictional and true-life accounts of persons with disabilities.

Brown, C. DOWN ALL THE DAYS (Stein & Day Publishers) and MY LEFT FOOT (Simon & Schuster, Inc.).

> The author has cerebral palsy and, of equal importance for the reader, is a spinner of Irish tales in the tradition of the greatest of Irish poets and authors. These are stories of growing up disabled.

Capt. Storm—P. T. BOAT SKIPPER (National Periodical Publications).

> This is a series of comic books portraying a person with a disability as a hero. Now out of print, these comic books may have limited appeal because of their war theme. However, the series is a piece of children's fiction that is unique in its characterizations. As the first issue states, "Introducing the battling sailor whom the enemy couldn't sink—even though he had only *one* leg to stand on!"

Drimmer, F. VERY SPECIAL PEOPLE (Bantam Books, Inc.).

> Have you ever gone to a sideshow at a carnival and wondered about the people who were the attractions? This book, as the cover states, "Reveals the real lives of human oddities— their loves and triumphs." Persons with physical deviations who have, for various reasons, exploited these deviations or have had them exploited by a gawking public are presented in this nonfictional account.

Freeman, D. CREEPS (University of Toronto Press).

> This play strips away the illusions of the sheltered workshop as seen by its employees.

Howard, M. ONLY HUMAN (The Seabury Press, Inc.).

> This is a fictional account of three teenage unmarried girls who become pregnant and the problems they encounter in dealing with their pregnancies and lives.

Term "more readable" from Porter, R. M. Books college students like to read about exceptional children. *Exceptional Children,* 1972, *39,* 240-242.

Jones, R. THE ACORN PEOPLE (Bantam Books, Inc.).

This is a nonfictional account of a summer camp counselor who learns that handicapped kids are, after all, just kids.

Kellogg, M. TELL ME THAT YOU LOVE ME, JUNIE MOON (Popular Books).

This story describes the ordeal of three young persons with disabilities—two men and a woman—who decide they can live together in the world of able-bodied prejudice.

Killilea, M. KAREN (Prentice-Hall, Inc.).

This is a true story by the mother of a child with cerebral palsy. A parent's point of view of living with a child with a disability is not to be taken lightly, as the reader will discover in this book.

Lund, D. ERIC (Dell Publishing Co., Inc.).

This is the true story, told by his mother, of a young man—an athlete—who dies of leukemia.

Neufeld, J. TWINK (Signet).

This short and easy-to-read novel pictures the life of a young girl with cerebral palsy, no speech, and other assorted problems, not the least of which seem to involve those who live around her.

Nichols, P. JOE EGG (Grove Press, Inc.).

This play digs very deeply into the emotional lives of parents who try to live with the fact that their beautiful daughter is severely involved with cerebral palsy.

Stein, S. B. ABOUT DYING and ABOUT HANDICAPS (Walker & Co.).

These two books are written for children. However, much as *Winnie the Pooh* is supposed to be for children, they are probably as well suited for adults as for the younger set. The pictures alone are worth the time and effort it takes to find and read these two gems.

Valens, E. G. THE OTHER SIDE OF THE MOUNTAIN (Warner Press, Inc.).

This book is about Jill Kinmont, who suffered a spinal cord injury in a skiing accident.

White, E. B. CHARLOTTE'S WEB and STUART LITTLE (Dell Publishing Co., Inc.).

Although the first of these two books for children deals with the subject of death, both books are statements about life. The first is the story of a pig destined for slaughter. The second is the story of human parents who have, for a son, a mouse named Stuart; this has some rather interesting parallels for parents of children who are disabled.

Wolf, B. DON'T FEEL SORRY FOR PAUL (J. B. Lippincott Co.).

This is a picture book story about a child who has had an amputation. It describes his everyday activities and his interactions with family and friends.

C Publications and educational materials sources

Publications

Accent on Living
P.O. Box 700
Bloomington, Ill. 61701

Achievement
925 N.E. 122nd St.
North Miami, Fla. 33161

Apropos
National Center on Educational Media and
　Materials for the Handicapped
The Ohio State University
Columbus, Ohio 43210

Closer Look
National Information Center for the
　Handicapped
Box 1492
Washington, D.C. 20013

*Directory of Organizations Interested in the
　Handicapped*
Committee for the Handicapped
People to People Program
La Salle Bldg., Suite 610
Connecticut Ave. and L St.
Washington, D.C. 20036

The Independent
2539 Telegraph Ave.
Berkeley, Calif. 94704

NAPH Newsletter
1162 Lexington Ave.
Columbus, Ohio 43201

Newsletter
Committee for the Handicapped
1028 Connecticut Ave. N.W. Rm. 610
Washington, D.C. 20036

Paraplegia Life
National Paraplegia Foundation
333 N. Michigan Ave.
Chicago, Ill. 60601

Paraplegia News
935 Coastline Dr.
Seal Beach, Calif. 90740

Rehabilitation Gazette
4502 Maryland Ave.
St. Louis, Mo. 63108

Educational materials sources*

Abbey Rents
Catalogue Sales
13500 S. Figueroa
Los Angeles, Calif. 90061

American Guidance Service, Inc.
Publishers Building
Circle Pines, Minn. 55014

Bureau of Education for the Handicapped
Office of Education
400 Maryland Ave. S.W.
Washington, D.C. 20202

Childcraft Education Corp.
20 Kilmer Rd.
Edison, N.J. 08817

Education Teaching Aids
159 W. Kinzie St.
Chicago, Ill. 61610

*Catalogues of teaching and therapeutic aids and materials are available from these sources on request.

Educational Activities, Inc.
P.O. Box 392
Freeport, N.Y. 11520

Flaghouse Inc.
18 W. 18th St.
New York, N.Y. 10011

Fred Sammons, Inc.
Box 32
Brookfield, Ill. 60513

Lansford Publishing Co., Inc.
P.O. Box 8711
San Jose, Calif. 95155

Learning Concepts
2501 N. Lamar
Austin, Tex. 78705

Library of Congress
Division for the Blind and Physically
    Handicapped
1291 Taylor St. N.W.
Washington, D.C. 20542

Love Publishing Co.
6635 East Villanova Pl.
Denver, Colo. 80222

Modern Education Corp.
P.O. Box 721
Tulsa, Okla. 74101

Skill Development Equipment Co.
1340 N. Jefferson St.
Anaheim, Calif. 92806

Special Learning Corp.
42 Boston Post Rd.
Guilford, Conn. 06437

Teaching Resources Corp.
100 Boylston St.
Boston, Mass. 02116

D Glossary

abduction Turning outward; movement away from the midline of the body.

acquired Not genetic; produced by influences originating outside the organism.

adduction Turning inward toward the midline of the body.

ADL Activities of daily living.

allergy Hypersensitivity to a specific substance that under similar conditions would be harmless to most people.

amblyopia Dimness of vision for which no organic defect in the refractive system of the eye has been discovered.

ambulate Act of walking.

amelia Congenital absence of a limb or limbs.

amputation Removal of a limb or limbs, or parts thereof.

anomaly Deviation from normal.

arthrogryposis Persistent flexure or contracture of a joint.

asthma Disease characterized by wheezing and coughing due to a spasmodic contraction of the bronchi.

Definitions have been selected or abridged from a variety of sources including:

> Dorland's *illustrated medical dictionary* (25th ed.). Philadelphia: W. B. Saunders Co., 1974.
>
> English, H. B., and English, A. C. *A comprehensive dictionary of psychological and psychoanalytical terms*. New York: David McKay Co., Inc., 1958.
>
> Holvey, D. N. (Ed.). *The Merck manual of diagnosis and therapy* (12th ed.). Rahway, N. J.: Merck & Co., 1972.

Note: No glossary of terms alone is sufficient for the development of a professional vocabulary. It is highly recommended that the reader acquire a good medical dictionary for reference.

astigmatism Refractive error due to defective surfaces of the eye.

asymmetrical Lack of similarity between corresponding parts on opposite sides of the body that are normally alike.

ataxia Lack of muscle coordination.

athetosis Continuous involuntary writhing motion.

atonia Lack of muscle tone.

atrophy Wasting away or decrease in size of a limb, organ, and so on.

aura Sensation before an epileptic seizure.

bilateral Referring to both sides of the body.

cardiac disorder Disorder pertaining to the heart.

cerebral hemisphere One of the pair of structures constituting the largest part of the brain in the human.

cerebral palsy Disorder of movement and coordination due to damage to motor areas of the brain.

congenital Present at birth.

contracture Condition of fixed high resistance to passive stretch of a muscle.

cystic fibrosis Inherited disease of the exocrine glands, affecting the pancreas and the respiratory system.

degenerative Alteration in form or function from better to worse.

diabetes melitus Metabolic disorder of the pancreas resulting in insulin insufficiency.

disability Objective, measurable lack of function or form.

Duchenne-type muscular dystrophy Most frequent type of muscular dystrophy, characterized by muscle weakness and wasting.

dysarthria Inarticulate speech, often associated with cerebral palsy.

epilepsy Central nervous system disorder marked by periods of unconsciousness; may also include involuntary muscle and organ activity.

etiology Study of the cause of a disease.

flaccid Weak, lax, and soft.

flexion Bending of a structure.

grand mal Epileptic seizure with loss of consciousness, lack of body control, and, possibly, incontinence; may be followed by deep sleep. There is widespread convulsive activity.

handicap Subjective or environmental limitations associated with disability.

hemiplegia Paralysis on one side of the body.

hemophilia Hereditary blood disorder resulting in insufficient clotting.

hydrocephalus Abnormal accumulation of fluid in and around the brain accompanied by enlargement of the head.

hyperglycemia Abnormally high level of glucose in the blood.

hyperopia Refractive error of vision: far-sightedness.

hypertrophy Excessive growth of an organ or its parts.

hypoglycemia Deficiency of glucose in the blood.

idiopathic Of unknown cause.

insulin Hormone produced by the pancreas, enabling the body to use sugar and other carbohydrates.

kinesthesia Sense by which muscular motion, weight, and position are perceived.

lateral Pertaining to the side.

Legg-Perthes (Legg-Calvé-Perthes) disease Degenerative disease of the head of the femur.

lordosis Exaggerated forward curvature of the spinal column.

myelin Fatlike substance forming a sheath around certain nerve fibers.

myelomeningocele Exposed sac containing neural elements of the spinal cord.

myopia Refractive error of vision: near-sightedness.

nystagmus Involuntary rapid, jerky movement of the eyeball.

orthotics Field of knowledge relating to orthopedic appliances and their use.

osteogenesis imperfecta Inherited condition in which the bones are abnormally brittle and subject to fractures.

paralysis Loss or impairment of function.

paraplegia Paralysis of the lower limbs or lower section of the body.

pathological Caused by disease, disorder, or abnormal condition of the organism or its parts.

petit mal Type of epileptic seizure with only a brief lack of consciousness.

phocomelia Developmental anomaly resulting in the attachment of the hands and feet directly to the trunk.

poliomyelitis Acute viral disease with possible flaccid paralysis of various muscle groups.

prognosis Prediction of the duration, course, and outcome of a disease or condition.

prosthesis Artificial substitute for a body part.

quadriplegia Paralysis affecting both arms and both legs.

remission Temporary abatement or cessation of the symptoms of a disease. Also, the time period during abatement or cessation.

RH factor Agglutinating factor present in the blood of about 85% of the population; causes antibody formation when introduced into blood lacking it.

rheumatoid arthritis Chronic syndrome characterized by inflammation of the joints.

rubella German measles; may result in congenital defects of infants born to mothers who were infected during the early months of pregnancy.

scoliosis Abnormal lateral curvature of the spine.

seizure Epileptic attack; changes in the state of consciousness, motor activity, and/or sensory phenomena.

spasticity Increase of muscle tension resulting in continuous increase of resistance to stretching.

spina bifida Developmental anomaly characterized by a defect in the bony encasement of the spinal cord.

strabismus Lack of coordination of eye muscles so that the two eyes do not focus on the same point.

syndrome Pattern of symptoms characterizing a particular disorder or disease.

tactile Pertaining to the sense of touch.

trauma Injury or wound.

tremor Involuntary quivering or shaking.

ventricle Any small cavity in an organ, such as in the heart or the brain.

Index